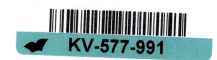
Nursing in action

Strengthening nursing and midwifery to support health for all

WHO Library Cataloguing in Publication Data

Nursing in action : strengthening nursing and midwifery
    to support health for all / edited by Jane Salvage

    (WHO regional publications. European series ; No. 48)

    1.Nursing – trends 2.Midwifery – trends
    3.Education, nursing – trends 4.Health for all
    I.Salvage, Jane II.Series

    ISBN 92 890 1312 5   (NLM Classification WY 16)
    ISSN 0378-2255

Cover design: Sven Lund
Text editing: Mary Stewart Burgher

World Health Organization
Regional Office for Europe
Copenhagen

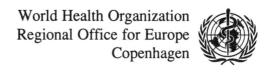

Nursing in action

Strengthening nursing and midwifery to support health for all

Edited by

Jane Salvage

Regional Adviser for Nursing and Midwifery
WHO Regional Office for Europe

WHO Regional Publications, European Series, No. 48

ISBN 92 890 1312 5
ISSN 0378-2255

The Regional Office for Europe of the World Health Organization welcomes requests for permission to reproduce or translate its publications, in part or in full. Applications and enquiries should be addressed to the Publications unit, WHO Regional Office for Europe, Scherfigsvej 8, DK-2100 Copenhagen Ø, Denmark, which will be glad to provide the latest information on any changes made to the text, plans for new editions, and reprints and translations already available.

PRINTED IN FINLAND

CONTENTS

Foreword

Promoting health, preventing illness, and caring for the sick and dying are age-old human concerns. Most people in need of such support will continue to find it among their communities, families and friends. In the formal setting of Europe's health services, however, nurses and midwives have important roles in health promotion, disease prevention, care and rehabilitation.

Nursing staff number about five million in our Region and account for a large part of the health care budget in every country. They are known by many titles and undertake a wide variety of roles and functions, from the central Asian feldsher delivering primary health care to the Scandinavian intensive care nurse; but whatever they are called, they are and will continue to be the backbone of any health service.

The profound changes in health care in our Region raise key questions for nurses. The issue is not whether they should change their practice, but how they will change it – and what role they will play in meeting the health needs of the future. Despite the differences, those five million workers face remarkably similar problems arising from their low status and from discrimination. They need active support at all levels to help them strengthen their contribution to health for all.

Above all, though, change comes from within, and nurses and midwives are already in the forefront of reform. In 1988, at WHO's European Conference on Nursing, the Region's nurses chose the strategy for health for all as the guiding star for the development of the profession. They set themselves the goal of creating a new kind of nurse. She or he will be an autonomous, skilled practitioner who can work alone or in partnership with other professionals to give primary health care in any setting. Her role will not be to serve another profession, but to inform, support and care for the patient and the community.

Creating this role, and ensuring it has the support necessary for it to be carried out, are formidable tasks. How can they be tackled? This book, the fruit of several years' work by experts throughout the Region, provides the starting point. It guides European nurses on what they can do, now and in the future, to shape their profession. While never losing sight of its vision, it gives practical advice on managing change, reforming education, establishing regulatory systems, and preparing leaders. It is my pleasure to commend it to all nurses and to all who support their aspirations – which means everyone who is working towards health for all.

J. E. Asvall
WHO Regional Director for Europe

Acknowledgements

This is a summary of the seven booklets in the Health for All Nursing Series, issued by the WHO Regional Office for Europe in 1991–1992. The content is largely unchanged but has been revised or reordered in some places to avoid duplication and ensure a logical sequence of presentation. The Nursing and Midwifery unit in the Regional Office pays tribute to the many nurses and midwives throughout the European Region who generously contributed their ideas, time, writing skills and money to create the original series.

Helpful comments on the original drafts were made by 27 European Member States. The following people wrote substantial sections of the text: Dr Fadwa Affara, International Council of Nurses; Professor Margaret Alexander, Glasgow Polytechnic, United Kingdom; Ms Anne-Marie Elliautou, WHO Collaborating Centre for Nursing, Lyon, France; Mr Colin Ralph, United Kingdom Central Council for Nursing, Midwifery and Health Visiting; Ms Muriel Skeet, international nursing consultant, United Kingdom; and Mr Steve Wright, The European Nursing Development Agency, United Kingdom.

Others too numerous to mention by name contributed ideas and working papers by taking part in a series of consultation meetings. These included the meeting of the steering committee chaired by Professor Margaret Green (Copenhagen, February 1990); the consultation hosted by the Centro Studi delle Professioni Infermieristiche, and chaired by Mrs Yvonne Moores (Turin, June 1990); the consultation hosted by the Hellenic Red Cross Society and the Hellenic National Graduate Nurses' Association and chaired by Ms Marjaana Pelkonen (Athens, June 1990); the meeting of the task force on curriculum review and reorientation co-sponsored by the Scottish

Home and Health Department and chaired by Ms Anne Jarvie (Edinburgh, December 1990); and meetings of the Commission européenne francophone des formations supérieures en soins infirmiers.

Financial assistance was received from the Centro Studi delle Professioni Infermieristiche, Italy; the Danish Nurses' Organization, Denmark; the Deutscher Berufsverband für Krankenpflege, Germany; the Gesellschaft Deutscher Krankenhaustag mbH, Germany; the Instituto de Salud Carlos III, Spain; and the Northern Nurses' Federation.

Special thanks go to Ms Elisabeth Stussi, former Regional Adviser for Nursing, Midwifery and Social Work, WHO Regional Office for Europe, for her vision and persistence in developing the Series, and to Ms Mary Stewart Burgher of the Publications unit in the Regional Office for her continuing interest in and assistance with the Series, and her help in preparing this book.

Finally, a note on terminology. The role, functions and even the title of the nurse and midwife vary enormously in the European Region. This book is aimed primarily at health personnel with a professional qualification in nursing, midwifery or equivalent. It is also relevant, however, to other groups such as feldshers, middle-level health personnel, and support workers who have a nursing function or orientation in their work.

Jane Salvage

Introduction

The Future of Nursing in the New Europe

The new Europe is an exciting place – so exciting that it is hard to keep up with the pace of change. The European Region stretches from Kamchatka in the east to Greenland in the west, and from Lapland in the north to Israel in the south. Recent political changes have brought the total of Member States in the Region close to 50. The European Region, then, is geographically huge and varied, and encompasses a rich diversity of races, cultures, religions and languages.

It is remarkable to reflect on how recently many changes have occurred: few people could have predicted, at the beginning of 1989, the rapid crumbling of the former regimes in central and eastern Europe. The destruction of the Berlin Wall, with all its symbolic significance, is now closely linked, politically and economically, with the moves of the 12 countries of the European Community towards greater unity. All this means new alliances, new conflicts and a new European order. It brings openness to change and experiment, but has also brought disaster, including civil conflict.

Nursing, of course, is not immune to these changes. The social, economic and political changes in every country influence health, health care and the practice of nursing, while nurses as citizens are influenced by their environment. New health needs are emerging in the Region, not least from the consequences of armed conflict. Infectious diseases, malnutrition, high maternal and child mortality, and physical and psychological trauma are just a few of the problems now ravaging our populations – problems that Europeans are more used to seeing in other parts of the globe. In addition, health needs that were always present but were denied by previous governments are now being openly expressed.

The countries trying to meet these old and new needs are short of money and often lack up-to-date knowledge or skills. The reform of the health care system is high on the agenda of many Member States, driven by poor standards of care, financial crisis, consumer dissatisfaction, dislike of centrally controlled structures, and ideological motives. Countries face the challenge of creating new systems that can meet demands more effectively at a time when the necessary human and financial resources are in short supply, and when the transition from centrally planned to mixed or market-based economies has reached a stage at which neither the old nor the new systems are working.

Nurses everywhere are facing huge difficulties, although these differ in degree. Countries are at different stages of development, and culture, politics, language and other factors make nursing in each country (or even each region) unique. Nevertheless, some universal themes appear to influence the development of nursing in every country. These may be summarized as power, gender and medicalization. All three are closely linked.

The first theme is power, or rather the lack of it. In no country of the Region do nurses play a full part in policy-making and decision-making at all levels of the health care system. Even in countries whose health ministries have large nursing departments, nurses must continually fight to ensure that their voice is heard. Many other countries, in all parts of the Region, have no nurse in a senior ministry position; in fact, the person in charge of nursing affairs is often a doctor. Health ministries alone do not change the world, but the strength of nursing at that level is important in both symbolic and political terms, and is a fair indicator of the formal power nurses have in a country. A lack of formal power at the top is likely to be reflected elsewhere, for example, in the absence of a nursing contribution to decision-making in the health care team.

Gender forms the second theme. In every country, women make up the vast majority of the nursing workforce; men rarely comprise more than 10%. Nursing everywhere is women's work, and shares the characteristics of other female-dominated occupations: low pay, low status, lack of recognition, poor working conditions, few prospects for promotion and poor education. As the United Nations has reported,

4

women constitute half the world's population, contribute nearly two thirds of its work hours, receive one tenth of the world's income and own less than one hundredth of its property.

Nurses suffer from this gender discrimination in their personal as well as their working lives. Most are obliged to work what has been called the double shift, coming home from a hard day in the hospital, clinic or community to spend their so-called spare time in caring for children, partners and elderly or disabled family members. In caring constantly for the needs of others, nurses often find that no one is caring for them. This is particularly stressful in countries where they must spend many hours obtaining necessities for their families. Simply keeping the family fed and clothed is thus a full-time job, and most men still regard domestic work and child care as a job for women.

The third theme is medicalization. Medicine dominates every European health system to a greater or lesser extent. Some steps have been taken to turn the rhetoric of the primary health care approach into reality, but in every country acute medical treatment receives the lion's share of prestige and resources. In the majority of countries in the European Region, health ministers, civil servants and senior health service managers are doctors. On the ward or in the community, nurses are often seen as medical assistants whose job is to carry out medical orders; the caring component of healing is invisible and undervalued. Of course, nurses do care for their patients and express their compassion through loving words and touch. In systems that do not acknowledge the importance of the caring role, however, nurses themselves undervalue it.

Very briefly, this is the backdrop for nursing development in Europe today. Clearly, these are times of both great danger and great opportunity. How are European nurses responding to the challenge?

Coming Together

Remarkably, nurses from all over the European Region had come together to share ideas and seek a common vision even before the world-shaking events of 1989. The previous year, nursing representatives from the then 32 Member States of the Region gathered in

Vienna, Austria for the first European Conference on Nursing. They brought with them the fruits of three years of discussions in meetings attended by thousands of people and held in 31 countries. As in all such conferences, there were plenty of arguments and disagreements, but an extraordinarily coherent and clear vision of the nurse of the future finally emerged *(1)*.

The greatest strength of this vision was that it was built, not on narrow professionalism, but on a broad understanding of nursing's contribution to improving people's health. It drew on the principles of the WHO movement to achieve health for all by the year 2000.

Following the Vienna Conference, the new role of the European nurse was further described and clarified in international consultative meetings, and a series of booklets (the Health for All Nursing Series) was produced to publicize the results. The mission of nursing was agreed to be helping people to determine and achieve their health potential, in their living and working environments. The nurse's chief functions should therefore be the promotion and maintenance of good health, the prevention of ill health, and giving care during illness and rehabilitation. The mission and functions of the nurse are discussed in detail in Chapter 1.

The key concept underlying the development of the nurse is the need to create a nursing role that is appropriate to people's health needs, rather than the needs of the health care system. It means a fundamental transformation of the nurse's traditional role as servant to the doctor and general dogsbody; she must be a well educated professional whose unique and distinctive contribution to health care is respected by all colleagues, and who is regarded as an equal partner in the health care team. The focus of her practice is working alongside the patient or community – jointly with other professionals, when necessary – to improve people's health.

It is the people themselves who will produce and maintain good health. All health care – whether it concerns people with acute illnesses, long-term disabilities or health-damaging behaviour that needs changing – can be effective only if it is is inseparably linked to the environment in which people lead their daily lives. In health care in general, as well as nursing in particular, the focus is therefore

6

shifting away from treating the individual person towards building relationships with families and communities.

Another strength of the new vision of the nurse is its consistency with modern nursing thinking. Nurses all over the world are producing descriptions of nursing similar to the one created in Vienna and putting them into practice in innovative projects, new curricula and everyday nursing and midwifery practice. Nurses can therefore feel both proud and confident that their colleagues share these ideas – an unusual and striking example of professional consensus.

The "Generalist Nurse"

The recommendations and the declaration that resulted from the Vienna Conference (Annexes 1 and 2, respectively) were comprehensive, addressing practice, management, education and research. The concept that received the most attention, however, was that of the "generalist nurse". The fourth recommendation calls for change in all basic programmes of nursing education to produce generalist nurses able to function in both hospital and community, with all specialist knowledge and skills subsequently acquired to be built on this foundation.

On the surface there seemed little to disagree with in this. Problems arose, however, in applying the recommendation in countries. Did it imply, for example, that basic or first-level training programmes to prepare psychiatric nurses, paediatric nurses or midwives should be phased out, and that these and similar courses should be subsumed in one broad programme giving a common foundation? In fact, the imposition of a strict blueprint for nursing is neither feasible nor desirable. Each country must find the solution most appropriate to its health needs. The WHO position statements on nursing, produced by a wide cross-section of international nursing experts, are intended to provide guidance and ideas rather than instruction.

The choice of the term generalist was never intended to place the generalist nurse in opposition to, or in preference to, the specialist. Rather, it was intended to indicate the need for a sound, broad-based basic education in nursing with a strong emphasis on primary health care. It does not imply that the nurse prepared in this way will never need to deepen her knowledge and skills in cancer care, primary health care, mental health or other aspects of nursing. Such is the richness of nursing knowledge today that no practitioner can ever complete her education with her first qualification. To avoid further misinterpretation, WHO has replaced the confusing term generalist nurse with the "health for all nurse".[a]

The issue of when and how to specialize in nursing is emerging as a difficult dilemma in all parts of the Region. When resources are so scarce, the question arises whether it is preferable to focus first on improving basic programmes, leaving specialist development for a later stage. Once again, local circumstances, along with an assessment of the real impact of each option, must guide the choice. Whatever choice is made, WHO can play an important role in preventing the duplication of effort by using a consensus of expert opinion to provide general frameworks and guidelines. Each country, health service or nursing school can adapt these to its own circumstances and needs. The experience gathered from many people and situations can be used to help minimize problems and to find solutions and models of good practice.

Nursing in Action

Helping to make such guidance available to countries is one of the major tasks of the Nursing and Midwifery unit in the WHO Regional Office for Europe. The unit also assists countries by recruiting experts to provide technical assistance on a variety of issues. The impetus of the Vienna Conference is continued at the international level through the WHO Nursing in Action project, which is based on the European six-year plan for nursing drawn up by the unit following the Vienna Conference.

---

[a] This summary uses current WHO terminology wherever possible. Many definitions of terms can be found in *Glossary of terms used in the "Health for All" Series No. 1–8* (Geneva, World Health Organization, 1984 ("Health for All" Series, No. 9)) and *A guide to WHO terminology for the European Conference on Nursing* (Copenhagen, WHO Regional Office for Europe, 1988 (document)).

The Nursing in Action project has two main foci: nursing leadership and nursing practice. In 1989 the World Health Assembly passed a resolution (WHA42.27) on strengthening nursing and midwifery in support of strategies for health for all, urging Member States to:

> encourage and support the appointment of nursing/midwifery personnel in senior leadership and management positions and to facilitate participation in planning and implementing the country's health activities.

This emphasis on nursing leadership was also evident in the follow-up resolution (WHA45.5) passed by the Assembly in 1992 (Annex 3).

This recognition of the importance of nursing leadership was endorsed several times in recent years at meetings of nurses and midwives organized by WHO. The participants repeatedly recommended that WHO continue to strengthen the network of nurses in senior positions in ministries of health, to facilitate both the exchange of ideas and information and the development of leadership skills. The need is great. As mentioned, although nurses are the largest group of health care providers, their contribution to policy-making in health and health care at all levels is underdeveloped.

In addition, greater expertise is needed in formulating nursing policy in line with the goals of health for all and in responding to rapid social and political change. Real, lasting progress in nursing will be impossible unless each country (and indeed each hospital, school and primary health care team) has its own clear, achievable action plan. Such a plan should be based on a vision of the goal, and then set out the concrete steps needed to realize the vision. Without such a plan, especially at a time of competing demands and limited funds, nurses will continue to drift, unable to establish priorities or take control of their future. They must learn how to set priorities and work towards their goals in an assertive and active way, instead of waiting for instructions from others. Leadership is therefore very important, although it may seem a remote concern to nurses working every day in communities and hospitals.

The second component of the Nursing in Action project focuses on the development of nursing practice. Nurses in all Member States give priority to improving the quality of practice. Key tasks here include developing innovative services, adopting the primary health care approach, becoming more sensitive to the needs of service users, and looking more closely at questions of effectiveness and efficiency. This will help nurses to create health care systems that are appropriate, equitable and committed to health for all principles.

In this part of the project, WHO helps nurses to share experience and ideas about nursing practice development. There is a great need to collect information on good practice, so as to discover the most effective nursing actions, and to disseminate the knowledge (not least so that nurses give concrete evidence of the importance of their contribution to health care). The Nursing and Midwifery unit is establishing a database of projects on good practice, in partnership with the European network of WHO collaborating centres for nursing.

Prospects

A great deal of exciting activity is taking place in nursing development in Europe, encouraged by WHO and many other organizations. But how well equipped are nurses to meet the challenges of the new Europe? Although these challenges are daunting, nurses face them with tremendous energy and enthusiasm. This is perhaps the most striking and praiseworthy value shared by nurses: altruism, or the pursuit of ideals beyond personal gain.

This introduction focuses on some of the problems faced by European nurses. What unites nurses across the European Region, and indeed across the globe, is stronger than what divides them. This summary of the Health for All Nursing Series is intended to help and inspire nurses to even greater efforts in pursuit of health for all.

1

Policies and principles

The WHO Context

In 1977, the Thirtieth World Health Assembly adopted two important resolutions. The first was the historic resolution WHA30.43 stating that:

> The main social goal of governments and WHO in the coming decades should be the attainment, by all citizens of the world, by the year 2000, of a level of health that will permit them to lead a socially and economically productive life.

The goal described in this resolution is now popularly known as "health for all by the year 2000". The second was resolution WHA30.48, which recognized the importance of nursing and midwifery personnel in primary health care, and requested Member States to study their roles and functions, and to plan for a rational increase in their numbers in accordance with country needs for primary health care.

Then followed a series of attempts to develop a new approach to health and health care, the most dramatic being the Declaration of Alma-Ata *(2)*. The Declaration marked a turning point in the programming for community health – nationally and internationally. It gave governments and health professionals broad directives for the shaping of education, practice and research in primary health care. Member States formulated their national strategies for health for all, and then regional and global strategies were worked out.

The global strategy for health for all by the year 2000 *(3)*, adopted by the Thirty-fourth World Health Assembly in 1981, is an expression of individual and collective national responsibility and a description of ways and means by which WHO can support it. The global strategy pays special attention to the training of health personnel.

Ministries of health and other ministries and educational bodies concerned, such as ministries of education, will review training in the light of projections for the number, types and quality of the different categories of health worker required. Such training will take account of the role of health workers in supporting individuals and families to provide self-care. They will make all efforts to introduce the necessary reforms in faculties of medicine, health sciences and other relevant training institutions, so that, in addition to their technical training, health personnel will become involved with the philosophy of health development as defined in the Declaration of Alma-Ata and in this Strategy.

In addition, the European Region formulated its own strategy calling for a fundamental change in countries' health development. It outlined four main areas of concern: lifestyles and health, risk factors affecting health and the environment, the reorientation of the health care system, and the political, management, technological, personnel, research and other support necessary to bring about the desired changes. The strategy also called for the formulation of specific targets to support its implementation.

Thus a new era in health development was inaugurated. The Member States agreed not only to intensify their efforts to improve health but also, in a spirit of international solidarity, to share their experiences and progress with other countries within the framework provided by WHO. Six guiding principles underline the 38 regional targets *(4)*.

- Health for all implies *equity*. This means that the present inequalities in health between countries and within countries should be reduced as far as possible.

- The aim is to give people a positive sense of health so that they can make full use of their physical, mental and emotional capacities. The main emphasis should therefore be on *health promotion* and the prevention of disease.

- Health for all will be achieved by people themselves. A well informed, well motivated and actively *participating community* is a key element for the attainment of the common goal.

- Health for all requires the coordinated action of all sectors concerned. The health authorities can deal only with a part of the problems to be solved, and *multisectoral cooperation* is the only way of effectively ensuring the prerequisites for health, promoting healthy policies and reducing risks in the physical, economic and social environment.

- The focus of the health care system should be on *primary health care* – meeting the basic health needs of each community through services provided as close as possible to where people live and work, readily accessible and acceptable to all, and based on full community participation.

- Health problems transcend national frontiers. Pollution and the trade in health-damaging products are obvious examples of problems whose solution requires *international cooperation.*

Meanwhile, the Nursing and Midwifery unit of the WHO Regional Office for Europe had already begun to prepare a study on nursing care, working from the premise that such care must be based on people's expressed and perceived needs and on sound scientific principles. The study's main finding was the need to redirect nursing practice in the light of the 38 regional targets *(5)*. It was proposed, therefore, that the unit organize discussions throughout the Region of the changes required in nursing practice, education, research and legislation. As mentioned, WHO acted as a catalyst by convening the first European Conference on Nursing, held in Vienna in 1988. Before this, numerous local and national discussions – involving representatives of international governmental and nongovernmental organizations, as well as 155 000 European nurses – raised awareness of the need for reorientation of practice and education.

The conference participants recommended that innovative nursing services be developed to focus on health rather than disease (Annex 1). In keeping with the European policy for health for all, the nurse's practice should be based on the primary health care approach. The Declaration of Alma-Ata *(2)* defined primary care as:

> essential health care based on practical, scientifically sound and socially acceptable methods and technology made universally accessible to individuals and families in the community through their full participation and at a cost that the community and country can afford to maintain at every stage of their development in the spirit of self-reliance and self-determination.

Put simply, these principles mean that health care services should be equally accessible to all. There should be maximum individual and community involvement in the planning and delivery of health care services. Care should focus on disease prevention and health promotion rather than cure. Technology should be used appropriately; that is, methods, procedures, techniques and equipment should be scientifically valid, adapted to local needs and acceptable to both users and the people on whom they are used.

Health care should be regarded as only a part of total health development. Other sectors, such as education, housing and nutrition, are all essential for the achievement of wellbeing. Within this framework the essential elements of a primary health care service are: education on prevailing health problems and methods of preventing and controlling them, the promotion of a safe food supply and proper nutrition, the provision of safe water and basic sanitation, maternal and child health care (including family planning), immunization against the major infectious diseases, the prevention and control of locally endemic diseases, the appropriate treatment of common diseases and injuries, and the provision of essential drugs.

According to the Declaration of Alma-Ata, these fundamental principles and elements of primary health care constitute a conceptual frame of reference that affects not only the planning, organization and delivery of health care, but also the professional education and training of those who deliver it (2). Nursing and midwifery practice should therefore focus on:

- promoting and maintaining health and preventing disease;
- involving individuals, families and communities in care and making it possible for them to take more responsibility for their health;
- working actively to reduce inequities in access to health care services and to satisfy the needs of whole populations, especially the underserved;
- multidisciplinary and multisectoral collaboration;
- assurance of the quality of care and appropriate use of technology; and

–   the restructuring, reorientation and strengthening of basic pro-
    grammes of nursing education needed in order to produce
    nurses able to function in this way in both hospital and commu-
    nity.

The participants at the Vienna Conference also expressed the need
for urgent action by governments and national health decision-makers
to help nurses make the changes required, and drew up a declaration to
express their commitment (Annex 2). These events gave rise to the
next phase of the nursing programme in the Regional Office, the
Nursing in Action project. This is intended to help Member States to
develop nursing programmes that provide services more appropriate to
people's needs and ensure the evolution of nursing as an attractive and
satisfying career.

The Nurse's Mission and Functions

The mission of nursing in society is to help individuals, families and
groups to determine and achieve their physical, mental and social
potential, and to do so within the challenging context of the environment in which they live and work. This requires nurses to develop and
perform functions that promote and maintain health as well as prevent
ill health. Nursing also includes the planning and giving of care during
illness and rehabilitation, and encompasses the physical, mental and
social aspects of life as they affect health, illness, disability and dying.

Nurses ensure the active involvement of the individual and his
or her family, friends, social group and community as appropriate in
all aspects of health care, thus encouraging self-reliance and self-
determination. Nurses also work as partners with members of other
professions and occupations involved in providing health and related
services.

Nursing is both an art and a science that requires the understanding
and application of the knowledge and skills specific to the discipline.
It draws on knowledge and techniques derived from the humanities and
the physical, social, medical and biological sciences.

The nurse accepts responsibility for and exercises the requisite
authority in the direct provision of nursing care. She is an autonomous

practitioner accountable for the care she provides. She has a responsibility to assess her personal needs for continuing education in management, teaching, clinical practice and research, and to take action to meet those needs.

The functions of the nurse derive directly from the mission of nursing in society. These functions remain constant, regardless of the place (home, workplace, school, university, prison, refugee camp, hospital, primary health care clinic or other site) or time in which nursing care is given, the health status of the individual or group to be served, or the resources available. Further, the functions should be reflected in the legislation governing nursing in each country.

Four functions

Four major functions are summarized here. The first is providing and managing nursing care, whether promotive, preventive, curative, rehabilitative or supportive, to individuals, families or groups. This is most effective when it follows a series of logical steps known as the nursing process:

- assessing the needs of the individual, family, group or community, and identifying the resources required and available to meet them;

- identifying the needs that can be met most appropriately and effectively by nursing care and those that should be referred to other professionals;

- ranking the health needs that can best be met by nursing care in order of priority;

- planning and providing the nursing care required;

- involving the individual (and where appropriate, family and friends) in all aspects of care and encouraging community participation (if relevant and acceptable), self-care and self-determination in all matters relating to health;

- documenting what is done at each stage of the nursing process and using the information to evaluate the outcome of the nursing care given, in terms of the individual, family, group or community, the nurse involved and the system within which the nursing care was given; and

– applying accepted and appropriate cultural, ethical and professional standards.

The second is teaching patients or clients and health care personnel, which includes:

– assessing the individual's knowledge and skills relating to the maintenance and restoration of health;

– preparing and providing the information needed at an appropriate level;

– organizing or participating in health education campaigns;

– evaluating the outcome of such educational programmes;

– helping nurses and other staff to acquire new knowledge and skills; and

– applying accepted and appropriate cultural, ethical and professional standards.

Acting as an effective member of a health care team is the third function. It includes:

– collaborating with individuals, families and communities, and other health workers to plan, organize, manage and evaluate nursing services as a component of the overall health services;

– acting as a leader of a nursing care team, which may include other nurses and auxiliary personnel, as well as users of nursing services;

– delegating nursing activities and tasks to other nursing personnel and supporting them in their work;

– negotiating the user's participation in the implementation of his or her care plan;

- collaborating with other people in multidisciplinary and multisectoral teams in planning, providing, developing, coordinating and evaluating health services;

- collaborating with other professionals in maintaining a safe and harmonious working environment that is conducive to teamwork;

- being actively involved in policy-making and programme planning, in setting priorities and in the development and allocation of resources; and

- participating in the preparation of reports to authorities and politicians at the local, regional or national level and, when appropriate, to the mass media.

The fourth function is developing nursing practice through critical thinking and research, which includes:

- launching innovative ways of working to achieve better results;

- identifying areas for research to increase knowledge or develop skills in nursing practice or education, and participating in such studies as required; and

- applying accepted and appropriate cultural, ethical and professional standards to guide research in nursing.

In view of these responsibilities and functions, the International Labour Office *(6)* has recommended that candidates for nursing training:

should have completed a full secondary education (which may vary from country to country), and have qualifications for admission that are equivalent to those required by a university or other institution of higher education.

Of course, individual countries will determine other desirable characteristics of candidates.

2

Changing
nursing practice

Change is part of the way of life of nursing today. Toffler *(7)* has argued that we live in:

> the roaring current of change, a current so powerful today that it overturns institutions, shifts our values and shrivels our roots. Change is the process by which the future invades our lives, and it is important to look at it, not merely from the grand perspectives of history, but also from the vantage point of the living, breathing individuals who experience it.

Thus nursing and nurses are part of the process of change, sometimes driving it, sometimes being driven by it. It leaves none untouched. Whether as participants in, progenitors of or reactors to change, nurses are involved. If nurses are accepted as part of wider social change, and indeed are expected to change their practice to meet the goals of health for all, then they must explore how this can be done. The knowledge and strategies that nurses use will largely determine the success or failure of their actions, the effects on them as a group and as individuals, and ultimately the effects on patients, communities and populations.

Nurses do not seem to have a history of managing and controlling change, yet this professional group has great potential. About five million people work in nursing jobs in the WHO European Region. They work in every conceivable health setting, come from a wide range of educational and social backgrounds, and in their professional and personal lives have contact with every section of the population. They already act as agents for change, often without recognizing it. Whether reviewing the way they organize their work, helping a family at home, teaching a patient with diabetes to change her lifestyle, or carrying out a quality survey, nurses are actively involved in change, wherever they work and in almost everything they do. Change is so big a part of the nurse's role that nurses often underestimate its significance, and thus may miss opportunities to improve its planning and organization.

To some extent this reflects a tendency in the profession to undervalue what nurses do. Dismissing nursing as caring, common sense or a menial job can hide its intricacy and value. Nursing becomes part of the scenery for the stage on which the grander and more exciting health acts (the technological advances and medical breakthroughs) are played out. The fact that most nurses are women reinforces this tendency. In a culture that gives the greatest status to the actions and values of men, women's work may be dismissed or ignored. Further, women's work is not seen to include working for change.

There is no evidence to suggest that nurses always and naturally resist change. In fact, nurses appear to engender a huge amount of change despite the obstacles. The health visitor who works with a family to improve the nutrition of the children, the midwife who prepares a mother and father for the birth of their child, and the hospital nurse who helps a patient to adjust to disability are all working in their own ways to produce change. Similarly, many nurses work for change as individuals in professional, social and political organizations.

How change is introduced is important. Resistance appears to be strongest when nurses feel change is forced on them. The many examples of this in the history of nursing include the development of the nursing process, which was often undermined because nurses felt that they were being pushed into change against their will. Attempting to bring about change by the use of power – by those at the top on the ranks below – is risky.

A crucial factor in avoiding resistance and creating acceptance appears to be the degree to which nurses themselves can determine the progress of change. This requires knowledge and skill, combined with the opportunity to participate in and control the change process.

Unfortunately, certain knowledge and skills that nurses need in order to take the lead in innovation – to be "change agents" – are not always readily available to them. Personal growth and awareness, communication skills and assertiveness are not included in all nursing education curricula. Indeed, it could be argued that the people in power in health organizations rarely encourage these qualities in nurses. Consider the implications if every nurse in Europe were an assertive, aware and skilful change agent! Because most of these agents would be women, the effects would reach far beyond nursing and health care to society as a whole.

Nurses may sometimes be denied opportunities for development because certain powerful individuals and groups fear the consequences. Further, the culture of nursing hinders change in some respects. Martin's research *(8)* emphasizes that the resources available, the working environment, the prevailing management and leadership style, and educational opportunities have equally important parts in determining the success of nurses as change agents. Nurses have a complex position in health care and in society; the challenge is to define what they need in order to change their situation, and to empower them to fulfil their potential in the care of others.

Managing Change

Before embarking on change, nurses should reflect on their situation, to decide whether they possess the requisite knowledge, skills and resources to achieve their goals. The nurse's aim may be, for example, to help a patient to change his lifestyle by giving up smoking, to work with colleagues to reorganize care on the ward, or to use the results of a patient survey to change the way a clinic offers its services. No matter what the aim, all proposals for change demand certain prerequisites:

- an understanding of how the organization concerned works and who are the influential people in it;
- a knowledge of what resources are needed and how to obtain them;
- teaching, communication and teamwork skills;
- an awareness of personal abilities, strengths, limitations and knowledge;
- an awareness of the practicalities of the work situation and organizational priorities;
- time;

- a knowledge of how change is achieved, and the different strategies that can be used; and
- managerial and educational support.

Even managing what appears to be the simplest of changes is therefore fraught with potential difficulties; success depends on a great many factors.

This section points out some of the main elements and stages in the change process. The nurse's personal knowledge and skills are crucial. Knowledge of how change can be brought about is likely both to make the management of change much easier and to lead to success. This knowledge is as important to nurses as knowing the principles of preventing cross-infection or how to deal with a cardiac arrest.

Three approaches

A growing body of knowledge about the management of change is now available to nurses. This literature *(9,10)* shows three approaches to implementing change.

The first is the "power–coercive approach". This is a top-down method, in which people in authority instruct others to do things differently. It assumes that people obey the orders of higher authority, and it is usually accompanied by some sense of threat (such as the loss of a job or other punishment) if they do not. This approach is a common feature of military and hierarchical organizations, or those that rely heavily on bureaucratic control. In the health field, it is associated with rigid and institutionalized ways of delivering care. Unfortunately, this approach appears to inhibit initiative and creativity in the people who receive the orders. It also underestimates the ability of individuals and groups to resist proposed change, or to revert to old ways of doing things once the attention of authority moves elsewhere.

Second, the "rational–empirical approach" assumes that most people are guided by reason and self-interest, and that, given choices, they will act in the way that brings maximum benefit to all. This

22

approach is also somewhat top-down and authoritarian. It assumes that information and instructions tend to flow in one direction, from people with knowledge and power to those without. A simple example would be a nurse providing a group of smokers with much information and all the logical knowledge on why and how they should give up the habit. The rational–empirical style would expect the smokers to quit simply because reason should prevail.

This approach leaves open the possibility that the workers in an organization can be manipulated, perhaps cynically, by people in authority. It raises the question, in health care particularly, of what happens when the interests of the staff conflict with those of clients. Whether people will always act on the basis of reason is also open to doubt. Ignorance and prejudice can influence nurses' approaches to care, as shown, for example, by the fearful response of many nurses to people with AIDS.

Third is the "normative–re-educative approach". This style differs from the others; here change moves from the bottom up. It is based on the belief that people need to be involved in all aspects of changes that affect them, because they will accept and implement only the changes that fit into their values, goals and relationships. This approach accepts the premise that people can best achieve change by acting collectively, with maximum involvement of the people in the group. Because the group owns the process and outcome of the changes, it is more likely to accept and sustain them.

In the first two strategies, power lies in the hands of people with knowledge and authority. Both therefore carry the risk of resistance or rejection by people who feel that change has been forced on them. Of the three strategies, a growing body of evidence in nursing favours the normative–re-educative style; it is argued *(9,11)* that this is more likely to produce long-term changes in practice. The approach has been extensively used in some WHO Member States to foster changes in nursing practice, for example in nursing development units – centres dedicated to innovation, improvement and evaluation in practice. In these centres, practising nurses can determine their path of change and spread the results outwards into the wider health care system.

Responses to Change

Different roles and responses in the change process can be identified. Considering these can help nurses to predict the reaction to proposed changes in their own setting, and plan for them accordingly. Ottoway *(12)* describes three groups that deal with change in different ways.

The "change generators" are people full of ideas about what needs to be changed. They marshal the arguments, keep up the pressure and often carry things forward using charisma, passion and enthusiasm. Once a need for a change is identified, "change implementors" help to carry it through. Sometimes implementors can be brought in from other organizations to help facilitate the change. For example, a consultant could be employed to teach staff new skills.

"Change adopters" do not initiate changes, but accept them into their practice or are affected by the results. This group includes staff who incorporate new ideas into their daily work or the patients who are affected by them. While all three groups are agents for change, the term change agent tends to be reserved for the people who guide and help staff to introduce changes.

Rogers *(13)* suggests a similar division. The leaders of innovation may at first be in a minority. Some (the early adopters) follow the suggestions enthusiastically, some (the early majority) with a little more thought and consideration. A further group (the late majority) may be somewhat sceptical, but eventually embrace the changes. Another small group (the laggards) may put up considerable resistance, try to subvert the whole process and never change their practices.

While these ideas may help nurses to identify possible responses to change, they should be viewed with caution. People are rarely so predictable. Further, it is important to consider why people respond as they do. For example, laggards may be labelled as difficult or negative. Not all changes, however, are necessarily for the better. A nurse resisting a proposal to cut staffing levels may be seen as a heroine by some and a laggard by others. Much depends on the nature of the change proposed, how it is carried through and the personal beliefs and values of the people involved. Some colleagues may be set in their ways, but is this because they do not see the relevance of the change, feel excluded from the process or fear the consequences?

Keyser *(14)* discusses the usefulness of four strategies in different situations. He calls the first approach *telling*. This usually involves a combination of the rational–empirical and power–coercive approaches. Here people in authority tell the staff what to do and expect them to get on with it. Some have argued that this style is acceptable for people that have "low ability" or lack willingness to change. Sometimes it is used to deliver information until the staff have accepted the change and developed confidence. Then the level of supervision and control can be reduced.

The second approach, *selling*, corresponds with the rational–empirical approach. Convincing information is provided so that the new idea is more readily taken up. This is most effective where people are willing to change at the outset.

The third approach is *participating*, which is principally normative–re-educative. Here the participants themselves identify the need for change and choose the direction they will take. The fourth approach, *delegating*, is an extension of the participating style. It appears to be most appropriate for individuals and groups who have already achieved a self-directed approach to change. The change agent provides some support, but only when asked by those involved.

Key strategies

This discussion shows that certain key strategies make the successful implementation of change more likely. Although managers and educators can give valuable support to the work of the staff, it is at the level of practice, where nurses work with patients and clients, that change matters most and its effects can be most directly felt. A bottom-up approach, with change agents using a normative–re-educative strategy to work with staff and patients, therefore appears the more likely to produce real, lasting change in norms and practices (see Fig. 1).

Staff involved in the change process are more likely to be committed to it, because they feel a sense of ownership.

Fig. 1. Summary of key points in the change process

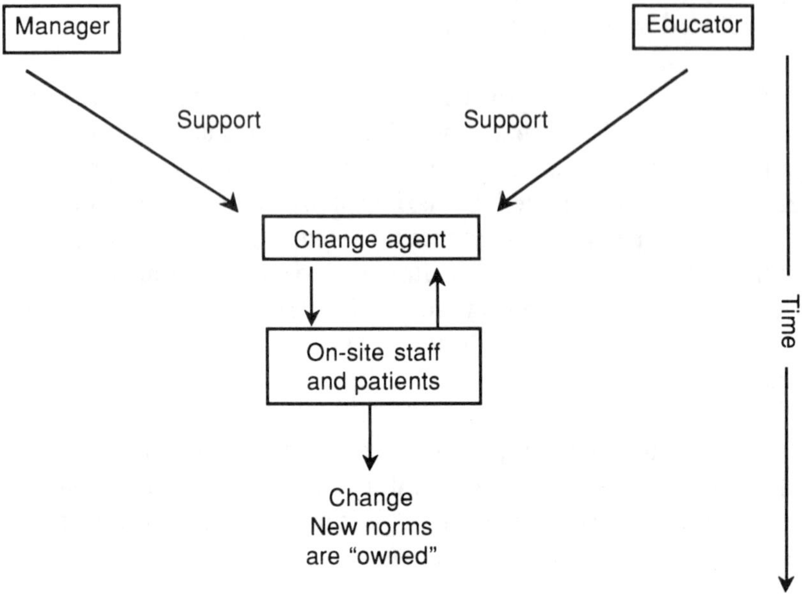

Manager

Educator

Support   Support

Change agent

On-site staff
and patients

Change
New norms
are "owned"

Time

Source: Wright (9)

Planning Change

Nurses can work as change agents in an enormous variety of settings. They can aim to change the behaviour of clients – individuals and groups – as well as colleagues, and be active not only within but also outside their immediate sphere of work.

While this chapter focuses on the knowledge and skills that nurses need to improve nursing practice, change in any sphere is much more effective if it is planned. Success does not depend only on having a bright idea and boundless enthusiasm; in fact, reliance on these alone is probably a recipe for failure. Enthusiasm and ideas need to be tempered with sober reflection and careful planning. This is not to say that planning will produce perfect results – it will not. Change by nature entails unpredictability. This can never be eradicated, even by the best laid plans. Nevertheless, good organization and planning can help to reduce potential risks and conflicts. This is especially important when nurses pursue changes that may affect vulnerable patients or clients.

Starting a cycle of change

Problem solving underpins the management of change, which has steps similar to those of the nursing process:

- assessing the situation
- planning (or deciding what needs to be done)
- implementing (or putting the plan into action)
- evaluating the effects and making changes.

Evaluating the effects of an action can lead to the reassessment and adjustment of the plan of action, so this process is often represented as a cycle of events (Fig. 2).

Fig. 2. Problem solving and the cycle of change planning

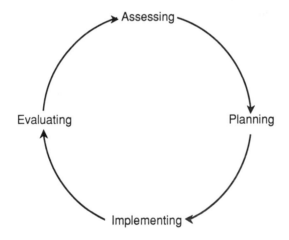

Ottoway *(12)* has refined this process in applying it to bottom-up change. It has seven steps. Agreeing on goals is the first step. The staff get together, examine the situation and decide that changes need to be made. The change agent has a key role in helping colleagues to think through their ideas and to make decisions about action.

Making a diagnosis is the second step. What is wrong? What do the staff want to change and why? Questions may need to be asked about how work is organized, who does what, what problems are encountered and why these occur.

The third step is designing the intervention. This involves mapping out what will be changed and how it will be done. The resources needed have to be determined, and the responsibilities of each member of the team identified.

Training comprises the fourth step. Staff may need training to learn new skills so that they can meet the demands of the changes.

The fifth step is implementing the intervention. The nurses put the plans into action and review them at intervals as the changes are under way.

Reinforcing new norms is the sixth step. Staff discuss the results of their work and identify clearly what has occurred. Improvements are pointed out, and praise and rewards for success are given.

The last step is replication. A review takes place of what has happened. Plans are modified if necessary and repeated elsewhere.

The following example illustrates these steps.

1. A group of nursing staff on a ward hold a meeting. Some people express dissatisfaction about the quality of meals available to patients. They decide to gather more information and formulate plans to improve the quality of service.

2. Further discussion and review reveal that patients' complaints about quality are only part of the problem. The staff do not organize the serving of meals very promptly.

3. The staff agree to change their work pattern near meal times, so they are free to serve the meals as soon as they are delivered to the ward. Two nurses agree to develop a questionnaire to gather patients' views. Another will approach the catering manager with the results and seek the advice of a dietician.

4. Conducting a patient survey and designing a questionnaire prove to be more difficult than expected. The staff seek the advice and support of a teacher and a researcher.

5. The staff start the survey, reorganize their work pattern and meet with managers, catering staff and dieticians.

6. At subsequent meetings, the staff report that patients are getting their meals more promptly. This is borne out by positive responses from patients. A thank-you letter is received from a patient. The catering manager has agreed to review the practices of the catering staff. The team leader congratulates the staff of the ward for the improvement they have produced. She promises further help in developing the survey tool and in providing staff with study leave to develop their skills.

7. After reviewing what has happened, the staff write a report on their experience. They circulate it in other wards, and attend meetings to share their experience. Nurses in other wards develop similar approaches.

A Change Culture

Readiness is another key factor. Why should a team or hospital seem to become ripe for change? This ripeness usually results from a combination of factors, such as:

- changing expectations of society and new laws and conventions
- changing aspirations and outlooks of nurses and other professionals
- changes in technology, medicine and health care
- local organizational changes
- objectives and decisions of local management
- new leadership patterns and the presence of change agents.

Any or all of these factors may combine to produce a climate for change. This climate does not affect all staff in the same way; some may be adventurous, others resistant. Indeed, success depends on people's willingness to take stock of their own situation, and their feelings about change and the part they can play in it. Just as external events and forces may affect the climate for change, so factors affecting motives and feelings determine each person's response. Thus each member of staff contributes according to her personal views and feelings.

The question is whether she:

- – sees the need for change
- – agrees with the change
- – wishes to support her colleagues
- – feels valued and supported at work
- – feels secure and supported in her personal life
- – sees change not as a threat but as an opportunity
- – sees possible rewards in the change, such as greater job satisfaction, better patient care or more pay.

People often see change as threatening when they feel cut off from decisions that affect their lives. This fact gives strong support for the bottom-up approach to change in nursing. Resistance is exacerbated when staff are unhappy at work or feel that their contribution is not valued. In addition, people with personal problems may be less willing to participate in innovation at work. Some senior staff resist change because they perceive it as criticism of past practices.

A work environment is supportive of staff when managers are helpful and accessible, learning is encouraged and staff feel reasonably rewarded for what they do. Such a climate is more likely to produce a culture that accepts change as motivating and beneficial. In such places, change becomes a way of life, a normal part of the day-to-day work that is accepted as commonplace and ordinary.

A Role for Managers and Educators

Nurses may be change agents at any level of organization. The change agent who works with nurses as part of the team has considerable advantages.

Many nurse managers and educators have very limited involvement in nursing practice. If they use their roles imaginatively, however, they can act as change agents by helping to create a climate that enables change to take place. They can support staff in the creation of a vision of a better future, which is the foundation of successful change. The manager often controls the budget, and so can ensure that resources can be made available when needed. Staff often turn to educators when they need further training. In supporting and enabling staff to pursue change, the manager and educator make a significant contribution to the climate. Indeed, they may be directly involved in managing the change, particularly if they have a direct clinical input. Alternatively, they can bring in new ideas and set new objectives to stimulate further innovation. Managers and educators should be cautious, however; practitioners can easily interpret encouragement from them as coercion and then resist it.

Many studies have shown how the manager can provide a milieu that either fosters or inhibits change. Through management and leadership style, the manager can influence the whole culture, which determines whether successful change is achievable. The manager is *(15)*:

> not divorced from more immediate operational matters. He/she is ultimately responsible for the allocation of resources of all kinds, for the organization of work and motivation of staff and probably for trouble-shooting and decision-making about contingencies. Undoubtedly there will be many other staff involved, and the degree of involvement may vary, but the ultimate responsibility lies at this level.

Thus, the nurse manager cannot remain aloof from the process of change, whether participating enthusiastically or standing on the side-lines. Managers and educators can influence change by both action and inaction. While the manager does not always have to be an active participant at the clinical level, her influence is still considerable.

Nurse experts working with WHO have already endorsed this view *(16)*. They saw nurse managers as essential to leadership in development, and called on Member States to:

> recognize the vital necessity of involving nurse leaders in the formula-tion and implementation of national health policies and plans, and ... encourage the creation, where they do not exist, of national/federal management positions from which nurse leaders may make this contri-bution.

The nurse manager therefore has a key role in the scheme of change. She can help to ensure that changes in one setting are not only fostered, but spread beyond the initial site. Manthey *(17)*, for example, suggests that an action plan be drawn up to promote wider organiza-tional change. The nurse manager at the highest level can help by setting up multidisciplinary steering groups. These not only support changes taking place in a small clinical unit, but can act cooperatively to ensure that the successes spread through the organization.

Piloting Change

When people make plans for change, they usually include a pilot scheme. This means choosing a specific site for the change, so that the results can be carefully scrutinized before the change is introduced elsewhere. For example, if a team decides to develop the nursing process, it may first agree on a trial period. This has several advantages. It allows other, similar settings to benefit from the team's experience. The problems encountered can be identified and future plans modified to take them into account. This allows other staff to save time, effort and resources. The change can be replicated elsewhere with the benefit of hindsight and with less risk of reinventing the wheel.

In addition, a pilot scheme carries the assumption that the change is on trial. This has many advantages. First, a pilot scheme allows more staff, including the more hesitant people, to feel involved; it does not demand the full commitment of every member of staff. This gives room for manoeuvre, time for staff to adjust, an opportunity for them to change their minds and a chance to demonstrate that the proposed change can work. It also allows the change to be adapted to take account of the unique qualities of the particular setting while maintaining its underlying principles. Further, introducing change in this way is a recognition of the need for flexible plans. People often feel more comfortable with change when they know that things can be modified. At the same time, giving staff time to create their own unique model reinforces their sense of ownership.

WHO nurse experts have encapsulated many elements of the pilot site approach in their endorsement of the development of demonstration projects *(16)*. The concept of a nursing development unit (NDU) also offers a model for a pilot site. NDUs are centres of specialist nursing practice dedicated to innovation and evaluation. They are committed to the development of nursing through the development of nurses, believing that the two go hand in hand. NDUs are also used as testing grounds for change. They try out new ideas, then share the results so that these can be taken up both locally and in a wider sphere. Pilot schemes with these characteristics are more likely to be successful, as well as to help to reduce resistance. Some further characteristics for piloting change can be identified.

1. The site chosen should be one at which the staff already demonstrate willingness for change.

2. Managers and educators should offer full support, including the provision of resources when necessary.

3. A reasonable amount of time should be allowed for making the change; it should not be expected to happen immediately. Staff should have the time to adapt, to work through difficulties and to set a target date for achievement.

4. The staff should organize the change themselves and spread it up through the organization, rather than the other way around.

5. The staffing levels, skill mix and other resources should be appropriate to the type of change envisaged. New equipment may be needed and, in some instances, long-term plans may be needed to change both the way resources and staff are deployed and the nature of the environment.

6. Training for staff development should be provided in advance when identified as necessary to support the change. At the same time, it should be accepted that training should also follow change. As new needs arise, additional development will be needed to sustain innovation.

7. The staff should make their own "contract" for change, deciding their roles, how long the pilot scheme will last and other matters.

8. A programme of evaluation should be built into the scheme.

9. The scheme should be designed for the unit involved; a ready-made package should not be transferred from somewhere else.

10. Plans for change should establish clear communication to minimize confusion and resistance. This would include: agreeing on

the frequency of meetings, ensuring the availability of assistance through papers and the visits of experts, ensuring that clear guidelines are given and responsibilities clearly assigned, giving feedback and making the team leader and managers available to give support.

11. A team leader should be clearly designated, and act as the principal change agent. The leader should have the expertise needed and work with the staff, offering encouragement, guidance and support.

The staff's feeling that things need to be done differently is an important step towards securing their commitment to plans for change. Sometimes staff recognize this need as they become aware of alternatives that might improve care. The feeling may also arise intuitively, or from the information gained by reading journals and research papers, attending courses, meetings or conferences, or learning about the results of patient satisfaction surveys. Whatever the cause, staff can begin to question and think anew about what they do.

It is difficult to say at what point this new equilibrium becomes the status quo. Change appears to have no real end, and the challenge for nursing is to develop a culture in which normal daily work includes reviewing and changing practices when necessary.

Conflict and Cooperation

Planning change and working collectively bring other advantages. Nurses working together towards common goals can have great strength, which the manager can reinforce with clear support. Inevitably, however, change brings some conflict. Many people find this challenging. It reinforces their desire to persist and stimulates them to be creative and questioning. Others find conflict stressful and demoralizing. Each person in a team responds differently, and many of the strategies thus far described would help to reduce conflict and engender a spirit of cooperation.

In some settings, the management structure is not responsive to change, or individuals or groups of staff resist very strongly. Changes sometimes provoke some staff to leave, which may disrupt the team, while providing openings for new staff who have new ideas and may support change. Change brings with it many volatile and potentially conflict-laden situations. A bottom-up strategy for change can do much to minimize the negative side of the process. Other useful tactics include:

- producing a well argued case for change, including both facts and a sound rationale (which can prepare the ground for change and indeed may contribute to a readiness to take part);

- avoiding confrontation;

- following accepted professional nursing guidelines and codes of conduct;

- ensuring maximum discussion of the proposed change among the staff involved (and with patients or clients, if they are directly involved);

- avoiding dogmatism, threats or the appearance of partisanship or self-interest (remembering that a willingness to negotiate is helpful);

- supporting individuals and groups of staff both at work and outside it (including not only study periods and opportunities for further development but also social events and the recognition that work should not be allowed to encroach on people's personal lives); and

- encouraging staff membership in a professional association or trade union (which can provide not only support in the event of major problems but also educational and networking opportunities).

Does Change Cost More?

Change always has costs. Some are personal: the time, energy and commitment of staff. Some comments in the previous section indicate how staff can be supported. It must also be accepted that any innovation has financial implications. These may include the time used by the staff or the new equipment needed.

An organization's lack of money may inhibit change. Indeed, in very difficult times, change may be the last thing people wish to think about. Nevertheless, this reinforces the view that nurses need to be able to present a good case for change. In the long term, a proposed change may actually save time and resources. Putting time, effort and resources into change can be seen not as a cost but as an investment in the future.

Building in Evaluation

Evaluation is the process of comparing results with the original plans for change. Did the plans work? If not, why not? What problems arose? What benefits emerged?

An evaluation strategy should form part of every plan of change, and can take many forms. It should include indicators to use in measuring what has been achieved, not least because others may be expected to replicate the changes at other sites. Change may affect the lives of colleagues and patients and can be costly; moral, practical and economic reasons therefore require the measurement of the effectiveness of what nurses do.

Change can be evaluated in many ways, but evaluations mainly fall into two groups:

- informal and formal
- quantitative and qualitative.

Informal methods require little structure or organization. Evaluation is often as simple as a view taken from a discussion at a ward or unit meeting to a nurse asking a few patients what they think of changes in the meals service. Such methods tend to be subjective, are often not documented and lack credibility if used to stimulate change elsewhere. Nevertheless, they provide managers and team members with a feel for what is happening, and can lead to changes in direction or the choice of more formal methods of evaluation. Informal methods can be helpful, provided their limitations are recognized.

Formal evaluation can be used to gather evidence that can more readily be used by others. It may be more expensive and time consuming, and involve a variety of methods of providing documented evidence. Sometimes the evaluation may take the form of a research programme, with the appointment of a researcher to oversee and carry out the work. Data may be gathered before, during or after the changes to enable comparisons to be made. The tools commonly used include questionnaires and interviews, gathering statistical information (for example, on discharge rates for patients before and after the changes), and keeping diaries. Although a full exploration of research methods is beyond the scope of this chapter, it is usually possible to choose one of a variety of methods to assess what is happening in the change setting. These methods have both strengths and weaknesses, and vary in complexity. When developing formal evaluation programmes, nurses need expert advice.

Quantitative methods of collecting evidence usually focus on hard data: facts and figures related to nursing or patient activities, such as sickness rates. Graphs, percentages, proportions and so on can be used to present the information and interpretations can be made from them. Qualitative methods focus more on the emotional and social components of the change. For example, quantitative research can number the patients who had care plans at the end of a trial period, while qualitative research would describe how the staff were helped to develop them, what attitudes and values arose, and how the staff actually used the plans.

Spreading the Word

Nurses often take part in exciting projects, but do little to tell others about their experiences. They can thus waste much time and effort in tackling problems that someone else has already solved. It is important to disseminate information on work that is completed or under way. Results, good or bad, need to be shared. Nurses can share their work by:

- producing written reports for internal and external use;
- joining a network of others with similar interests, or professional organizations that offer information sharing;
- accepting invitations to speak about their projects at meetings and conferences;
- producing texts of varying length and style for publication in journals, research bibliographies and elsewhere;

- giving information to the mass media (newspapers, television and radio);
- making tape recordings, including videotapes; and
- providing open days and study sessions on their projects (Fig. 3).

Even if none of these methods is used, word tends to spread. Relying on rumour or word of mouth, however, carries the risk of inaccuracy in the information that leaks out.

Fig. 3. Spreading the effects of change beyond the pilot site

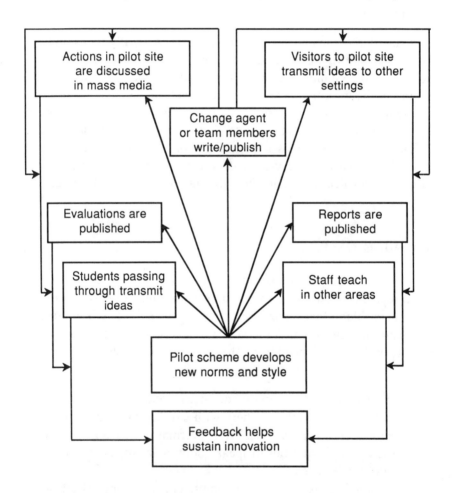

Source: Wright *(9)*.

Conclusion

Nurses are well placed to be change agents in the health care system and in society as a whole. Acquiring the knowledge and skills to manage change will make them more effective in this role. Nurses have often relied on heroines – charismatic and forceful leaders who drive change forward – but the scope for this model is limited. Thoughtful planning for change using a collective approach, with nurses working together for action, and a programme of managerial and educational support are much more likely to ensure long-term, meaningful changes in attitudes and behaviour.

Nurses need to seek the ownership of change, to learn how to plan it and to recognize the pitfalls and know how to avoid them. They need to share their knowledge and experience with each other, to keep up to date in their profession, to continue their personal growth and to develop their awareness. While they may be able to do this in advance of a specific change programme, the act of change, with all its conflicts, offers a great opportunity for learning and growth.

Nurses often set high standards for themselves, but they need to allow time for change to take place and to cherish achievements in the process of change, no matter how small. At the same time, nurses should also care for themselves. While being committed, energetic and passionate at work, they must also make space for their own pleasures, pastimes and friendships.

While change can be studied, prepared for and planned, it can never be simple and straightforward. In reality, it is rarely as linear and sequential as many of the theories mentioned here might suggest. There are limits to certainty. Volatility and unpredictability accompany change. Unexpected situations can arise and people can respond irrationally. The nurse who masters change is able to use a wide range of knowledge and techniques and adapt them to many different circumstances. Such a nurse is a potent force for change in health care, and an equal contributor to raising the quality of care for patients. Leaving aside issues of professional and personal growth, or the increase of the status of nursing, what really matters is that change improves the care of patients. The nurse who can change and improve practice gives valuable service to the wellbeing of others.

3

Developing
a regulatory framework

To survive, establish an identity, maintain integrity and bring order to its affairs, a professional group often seeks a regulatory system to bring consistency and control to its occupation and its practice *(18)*. The impact of regulation on an occupation can be pervasive and powerful. In nursing, regulation:

- in the form of admission standards, determines who is selected;

- in the form of educational standards, shapes nurses' capabilities;

- through the processes of registration and licensure, determines who will practise, defining, naming and certifying nurses to the public and employers;

- in the form of definitions of the scope of practice, other health and employment laws and a multitude of related rules and regulations, categorizes nurses and determines what they may do, where they may practise and what decisions they can make; and

- through systems of job classification, salary scales and promotion schemes, controls and distributes rewards.

In effect, regulation can determine the status and nature of nursing practice. It can enlarge or diminish nurses' capacity to perform to the best of their ability. It can increase or impede nursing's ability to respond appropriately to advances in knowledge and technology, and to changing health care priorities.

It is therefore necessary to ensure that nursing regulatory systems support efforts to move nursing in the direction described in the Vienna Declaration (Annex 2). Countries need to review their current regulatory policies and practices. Regulatory barriers, particularly restrictive definitions of the scope of practice and inadequate educational standards, have prevented nurses from maximizing their contribution to primary health care *(4,18)*.

This chapter addresses two areas related to the regulation of the nursing profession: a framework for a system to regulate nursing education and practice, and the relationship of regulation to nursing workforce planning.

Framework for a Regulation System

Basic concepts and dimensions of regulation

In essence, nursing regulation means bringing the practices of nurses under the control of some authority. Such control gives the authority the right and power to check, verify and determine limits and to exercise restraining powers to keep practice within those limits. This authority may be established by law, custom, convention or consensus *(19)*.

The nursing profession may be controlled by authorities outside it, that is, by external regulation. The most common and usually the most powerful is that applied by government through its power to make laws, rules and policies. Regulation that results from legislation is called statutory regulation.

In addition, authorities within the profession may regulate nurses and nursing. This self-regulation can occur at several levels – those of the individual practitioner, the work group, the health care or academic institution, the national nurses' association or trade union and the International Council of Nurses (ICN).

While the goal of external regulation, particularly statutes, is to protect the public, self-regulation goes beyond that point. It seeks to assure high-quality care while advancing nursing practice through the development of its skills and knowledge base. Thus, while statutes tend to define standards (for licensure, for example) at a general and minimal level, self-regulation is used to achieve a continuous improvement in nursing practice for the benefit of society. The formulation and continual updating of the standards for practice and education, which guide nurses in improving care, form an example of self-regulation.

Professional regulation has a number of dimensions. They influence decisions on the requirements for the efficient functioning of a regulatory system within a given context. These dimensions address:

- the purpose of regulation
- the nature of the regulatory authority
- the objects or entities to be regulated
- the methods of regulation.

Purposes

Regulation has numerous purposes, sometimes complementary, sometimes conflicting as the regulatory system tries to serve the interests of society, the profession and its members. These purposes range from assuring acceptable nursing care and protecting the public from unsafe practitioners to fostering the development of the profession, giving accountability, identity and status to practitioners, and promoting nurses' economic and general welfare.

For a coherent, effective and relevant system, the purpose of regulation must be explicit, because it will influence the decisions made in the other parts of the system. Who will have the authority to regulate what, or who will be regulated and what methods will be employed?

Nurses are essentially in the business of offering a service to society. The profession therefore has an obligation to ensure that the population receives an acceptable level of care. According to ICN *(18)*, the central purpose of statutory regulation should be to protect the public by ensuring competent and accessible nursing care. Benefits to the profession and the practitioners are secondary.

If regulation is intended to protect the public by ensuring that only qualified nurses practise and that their practice is safe and effective, the regulatory system must address at least *(18,20)*:

43

- the definition of the scope of nursing and categories of nurses;

- educational standards, such as admission requirements, curriculum content, learning experiences, faculty qualifications and educational facilities;

- measures to check the maintenance of practitioners' competence; and

- a mechanism for disciplinary action to deal with such problems as disability, misconduct and malpractice.

Nature of the authorities

Several authorities or agents may be involved in the process of regulation, particularly in setting standards and administering the system. ICN says that regulatory systems should recognize and incorporate the legitimate roles and responsibilities of interested parties – the public, the profession and its members, employers and other professions – in these tasks *(18)*. The roles, responsibilities and degree of involvement of the various parties differ between countries. The factors that may determine the level of involvement include regulatory traditions, political structures, public policy, the evolution of nursing, the dominance of other health professions and the level of representation of nursing in the regulatory process.

In most situations, however, four groups have regulatory responsibilities. First, the government can play a major role in regulating nursing through laws, administrative rules and regulations, and public policy. Legislation gives statutory recognition to nursing, defines the limits of practice, sets licensing standards and protects the practitioners' rights (for example, to perform certain activities or to the exclusive use of a title). In addition, the government is a major player in administering statutory regulation. It may do this directly or delegate its responsibility to another body.

Second, the profession plays a critical role in establishing and recommending standards for statutory regulation. Owing to its technical and interpretive expertise, nursing should also participate actively in administering governmental regulation, and represent its interests and those of its practitioners. Active and sufficient representation on the board or council administering the law is one way to do this. Finally, the profession has a fundamental duty to promote the growth of self-regulation.

Third, the practitioner has a regulatory function in practising according to established standards of care, codes of practice and ethics, and by taking steps to maintain her competence.

Fourth, the employer, through activities such as the development of employment requirements, institutional standards and quality assurance programmes, is an important agent of regulation.

Because the agents involved vary between countries, legislation on nursing education may be the responsibility of the education ministry, while the health ministry may regulate nursing practice. Alternatively, administrative responsibility for nursing regulations may be a joint function of both ministries or the sole responsibility of the health ministry. In a growing number of countries, the administration of acts on nursing practice is delegated to the profession itself through a statutory body (a body constituted by law and responsible for administering the law), most of whose members are nurses.

Objects or entities

The focus of control (the parties to be regulated) may be practitioners, educational programmes or service programmes. One or more of these may be regulated. The decision on what should be controlled and how to do it depends on the purpose of regulation and questions of feasibility, the adequacy of resources to administer the system and the availability of expertise. The regulatory system must be practicable and sustainable if it is to achieve its purpose.

Methods

After decisions are made on the purpose of regulation, the identity of the regulatory authority and the objects to be regulated, the question remains as to how regulation is to be carried out. What will the mechanisms and instruments be?

Mechanisms. Regulatory mechanisms vary according to the objectives of the regulatory processes. Self-regulation is receiving more attention as nursing evolves into a more autonomous profession. Registration and licensure are most frequently applied, however, for the statutory regulation of the individual practitioner. As they are the most frequently employed mechanisms, it is pertinent to explore how they differ.

Registration, if the term is literally applied, is the process by which people are assessed and given status on a register attesting to their ability (or qualifications). Registration entitles a person to bear a specific title. Although registration in nursing limits the use of a particular title to registered nurses, it does not usually limit practice to them. For this reason, it is called voluntary or permissive regulation.

Licensure, on the other hand, is a more powerful mechanism. It is the process that permits people with predetermined minimal competences to practise nursing. It is a mandatory or compulsory process and restricts practice to licensed individuals.

Relicensure or reregistration may depend on evidence of continuing competence. This may take the form of the completion of continuing education courses, documentation of active practice and even¡ re-examination. It has been argued that a mechanism to ensure competence throughout a nurse's career is necessary to protect the public *(18)*.

A further mechanism worth mentioning is accreditation or approval. It is used to regulate educational or service institutions and programmes. Accreditation or approval denotes that a programme or institution has met the minimum standards set by an appropriate statutory authority.

Instruments. To achieve control and consistency, certain instruments have been developed to judge the competence of practitioners and the quality of educational and service programmes. Instruments of regulation include standards, codes, validation measures such as examinations, references or recommendations, audits, performance reviews and disciplinary proceedings.

The effectiveness of regulation depends on the relevance of these instruments to its purpose. Standards of education and practice should be relevant to the type of practice required by current health needs, and evaluation methods should in turn be relevant to the standards. In addition, feasibility – the availability of resources and expertise – should influence the choice of the instrument eventually selected, if a system is to remain practicable.

A framework for statutory regulation

When the basic concepts and dimensions of a regulatory system have been explored, the identification of the basic requirements for a workable regulatory system for nursing follows. Three assumptions are made about such a system.

1. The nursing profession seeks greater participation in and control of the regulatory process. New roles for nurses entail greater autonomy in making clinical decisions and in managing and allocating resources. Regulatory systems should reflect this increased autonomy and emphasize the accountability of nursing to the public.

2. Demographic, epidemiological, political, economic and social trends in Europe are creating new health priorities that require changes in nursing. The regulatory system should be flexible enough to respond to changing health priorities and thus changing needs for nursing without losing effectiveness.

3. The central purpose of statutory regulation is to protect or benefit the public. In offering a service to the public, nurses have the obligation to ensure effective delivery. The public can be protected only if all who practise nursing are licensed. Because the public should not be expected to distinguish between competent and incompetent practitioners, the statutory regulation of practice is required.

Approaches to statutory regulation inevitably vary between countries. Certain features, however, encourage the development of relevant, consistent and effective statutory regulation, while permitting nurses a sufficient degree of participation in the formulation of regulatory policies and practices and in the administration of the system.

The following questions followed by discussion are used here to examine the issues.

Purpose

1. Do any of the statutory documents regulating nursing contain an explicit statement of purpose?

2. Is the protection of the public the primary purpose of the legislation?

3. Does the statement of purpose deal with the control of nursing practice and the control of educational preparation for that practice?

In considering the purposes of a law on practice, one should distinguish the control of education and licensing from provision for the social and economic welfare of the nurse. Factors such as good working conditions, pay and benefits are important, but they can be dealt with through other forms of legislation (such as labour, health and safety laws) and modes of action (such as negotiation).

Laws regulating practice should focus on the professional content of nursing and ensure that society has access to competent practitioners. Such legislation also gives legal recognition of nursing and protects nurses' titles and practice.

Definitions

1. Do definitions of the scope of nursing practice and categories of nursing personnel appear in the statutory document(s)?

2. Are titles clear and descriptive, identifying beyond doubt the nurse, nursing auxiliary or nurse specialist?

Statutes on nursing must contain a definition of the practice that they seek to regulate. Statements of the scope of practice define nursing and outline the boundaries within which the nurse operates. They may leave the nurse free to act to the limit of her judgement and ability, or restrict her to various procedures prescribed and supervised by others.

Such statements should be broad enough to allow flexibility in the use of nursing personnel, yet specific enough to provide guidance on the role and function of the nurse. A broad definition of the scope of practice does not require amendment when new functions appear. If necessary, functions can be defined more specifically in supplementary rules and regulations. These are more easily altered, since they are not required to pass through the law-making process. A broad definition also facilitates changes in the nursing role, particularly in primary health care, and promotes greater congruity of the legal with the real scope of practice. Further, it gives nurses authority to take up new roles and protects them from charges of practising beyond the law. WHO guidance on the mission and functions of the nurse (see Chapter 1) can help in drawing up such a statement.

It is important that there be only one definition of the scope of nursing practice and that the nurse be responsible for the range of care it covers.

Categories of personnel can be distinguished by defining the differences in their knowledge, roles, practice settings and levels of accountability. For example, if the concept of the nurse recommended in the statement of the mission and functions of the nurse is accepted, definitions of categories of nursing personnel will make it clear that the nurse is responsible and accountable for all nursing work, with nursing auxiliaries assisting under prescribed conditions (for example, according to standards for practice and under the direct or indirect supervision of nurses) and with the postbasic nurse specialist providing expertise in a particular field. Titles should clearly indicate who is the nurse, nursing auxiliary or nurse specialist. The word nurse should be reserved solely for people who are authorized by law to practise the full scope of nursing.

Administration of the law

1. Does the law provide for the administration of the regulatory system?

2. Who is responsible?

3. If administration is delegated to a particular statutory body, what is its composition and how is its membership decided?

4. What are its powers?

5. What degree of participation does nursing have in the administrative process?

Several patterns for administering acts on nursing practice can be identified. The most common is the creation of special nursing boards, councils or commissions. Another approach is for the ministry involved (usually the one responsible for health) to retain the responsibility of conducting the regulatory process through one of its departments, often one that focuses on nursing.

Ideally, nursing should have the responsibility to regulate itself through a statutory regulatory body, with nurses comprising a majority of the members and a nurse as its head. In addition, participating actively in selecting the members is clearly in the profession's interest. A combination of appointment, nomination and election procedures can be used to ensure that an appropriate balance is struck in the representation of interested parties.

The principal function of the regulatory body is to establish and implement standards of education and practice for nurses under the jurisdiction of the law. The power to make rules and regulations to supplement the main provisions of the law is important, as shown in the section on defining the scope of practice. If the proper procedures are followed, rules and regulations will have the force of law. The following important functions may be delegated to a regulatory body:

- implementing the law
- interpreting statutes and regulations
- making and enforcing rules and regulations
- defining nursing practice
- regulating through registration or licensure
- setting standards for education and practice
- maintaining a register of practitioners
- approving schools
- designating and regulating auxiliaries and specialists
- disciplining licence holders
- setting and conducting examinations
- creating committees to carry out functions
- assessing and collecting fees.

Standards

1. Are standards for nursing education and practice identified in the statutory document(s)?

2. Are the standards consistent with the health needs of the country?

3. How much does nursing participate in the process of setting standards?

Much regulation revolves around the preparation of the nurse for practice. A regulatory body therefore has an important responsibility to ensure that educational programmes are capable of producing the type of practitioner prescribed in the scope-of-practice statement. This goal is principally achieved through setting educational standards that are consistent with nursing practice as defined in the law and in supplementary rules and regulations. Educational standards should not be limited to setting curriculum requirements. The neglect of other factors – such as the organization of the school of nursing, faculty qualifications and learning and clinical resources – indicates inadequate regulation. Areas appropriate for setting educational standards include *(21)*:

- requirements for schools of nursing, covering their administration, direction, faculty qualifications, teacher–student ratios and facilities;

- requirements for clinical learning sites, including standards of care and the satisfactory control and supervision of students;

- requirements for admission to education programmes, such as candidates' general education, qualifications, age and health;

- the curriculum, including its length, objectives, content, teaching and learning methods, assessment and evaluation; and

- requirements for eligibility for registration or licensure, such as the completion of an approved educational programme or of a "return to nursing" course.

Standards for practice can focus on the nurse, and nursing practice and its setting. Statutory regulatory systems tend to focus on the nurse.

They are concerned with standards that relate to the nurse's behaviour in her professional role: competence for the entry into practice, accountability, the maintenance of competence and ethical behaviour. Many instruments – examinations and other evaluation methods, codes of ethics, conduct and practice, guidelines and criteria for demonstrating continuing competence – may be employed.

Again, the nursing profession should play the primary role in proposing standards for governmental regulation. It can do this by seeking adequate representation on the regulatory body, by establishing programmes for developing and testing standards, and by participating in the quality assurance programmes of the government or institutions.

Guidelines on framing the legislation

The guidelines that follow summarize and organize the material already discussed. They are flexible enough to permit the development of nursing practice based on primary health care, they provide nurses with sufficient autonomy in their practice, and they make nursing accountable to the public for the quality of nursing care.

Two levels of regulation can usually be identified in a regulatory system. The law accords legal recognition and sets up a system to regulate nursing; it is supplemented by rules and regulations. The specificity of the law and the rule-making power accorded to the regulatory body determine the flexibility of the system. A specific law (which, for example, incorporates details of the nursing curriculum and sets the level of registration fees) usually restricts flexibility, since changes would require amendment of the law.

The law should:

- have a statement of purpose;
- define the scope of nursing practice and the categories of personnel to be regulated; and
- set up a regulatory body and specify its composition, the method of selecting its members, its powers and functions, and its resources to conduct affairs.

Through its powers to make rules and regulations, the regulatory body should:

- identify the functions or activities of the nurse
- define standards for education and practice
- develop procedures and rules for carrying out functions.

These are the minimum requirements to meet the conditions described at the beginning of this chapter. Conditions in each country (particularly the organization of its health and nursing systems, regulatory traditions and the stage of evolution of nursing) will inevitably influence the final form of the statutory system. It is hoped, however, that these guidelines will help nurses to examine their current system of statutory regulation and correct the features that keep nurses from contributing fully to the development and implementation of primary health care.

Regulation and Workforce Planning

Development of a registration system

A national registration system is central to an effective regulatory system, and can bring order and consistency to standards for nursing education and practice. It can also provide data for the better planning and allocation of nursing resources. The registration system can serve these purposes in four ways:

1. By establishing criteria for registration, it sets a standard of education that a person must meet to be registered as a nurse.

2. By restricting the practice of nursing to people who are registered, it guarantees a minimum level of competence in those providing nursing care, and helps to maintain a collective standard for the profession as a whole.

3. It provides a base for the further development of the profession beyond the initial (or basic or preregistration) level.

4. It provides an opportunity to maintain, at a central point, certain records on nurses within the jurisdiction of the registration system.

The terms registration and licensure have already been introduced, but it is important to explore them further. Registration literally means that a person's name has been entered in a register or record. In a nursing register, the entry attests to the satisfactory development of the person's skills and knowledge following a course of nursing education that leads to the award of a diploma or degree. Registration should also ensure that the title of registered nurse is applied only to the people with the relevant education and qualifications. Registration therefore confers the right to practise as a professional nurse, and a regulatory system can prevent unqualified people from practising.

Registration can do more than merely maintain a simple record of people's names and dates of qualification. An effective registration system has a mechanism to update records. This may be linked to a regular requirement for continuing education or the demonstration of competence, before a further period of registration – and therefore practice – is permitted. In a number of countries, this aspect of registration is known as licensure, and this term is used here for consistency. Licensure is a powerful mechanism that permits people to continue practising nursing as long as they continue to meet requirements of the registering (or the regulatory) body *(18)*.

If registration and licensure confer the right to use the title of registered nurse and thus permit practice, it follows that the title and right to practise may be withdrawn if a registered person ceases to meet standards or harms patients. Mechanisms must be in place to protect the public by dealing fairly and effectively with both failure to meet standards and professional misconduct. Such arrangements form a major element of a regulatory system.

The purpose of a register must be clearly identified and the nature of the information to be recorded clearly determined.

The register as a record

As a simple, central record, the register must contain the name, age, sex, address and qualifications of each qualified person. The record may also show the educational qualifications of entrants to nursing education; these are likely to be useful for future research (for example, to compare the qualifications of people entering nursing education with their later examination results). To allow the use of such information, an index must be made of all students who enter nursing education programmes, so that the results of examinations can be analysed and interpreted for the development of selection criteria.

For the register to be complete, all students must be indexed and all those who successfully complete nursing education must be registered. This means that all schools and colleges of nursing must be approved. In many countries, success in examinations may be only one criterion for registration; confirmation of good character, for example, may also be required. In the few countries where, for historical reasons, more than one level of professional nursing education is still provided, the same form of record is required for each level, and a separate part of the register should be reserved for each. In addition to recording the basic or preregistration course of education, the register may also record subsequent postbasic or post-registration qualifications.

Entries to a register of this sort are usually not amended unless the register is part of a regulatory system that includes mechanisms for the regular issuance of licences to practise and for the removal of names in case of proven professional misconduct. Without this updating mechanism, a register is only a list that quickly becomes limited and out of date. Nevertheless, by restricting the use of the title of registered nurse, such a register ensures that nurses who practise are qualified to do so.

The register as a live record

Special mechanisms are required to convert a register into an up-to-date or "live" record. As entries in the register all relate to particular people, the most effective means of gathering up-to-date information is to maintain regular contact with them.

Some countries require nurses to obtain a licence to practise at regular intervals – usually every one, two or three years. Licensure therefore has immediate benefits. It provides an opportunity for regularly updating the entries in the register and for regular contact between the regulatory body and the members of the profession. It also provides a mechanism that links continuing education and competence with the registration system. Under this system, the registered person usually pays a fee to the regulatory body. As well as providing funds for the regulatory body, such fees cover the cost of changing the register entries.

One overriding principle of a live register is that the nature of the regulatory system must be directly related to the development of the profession. In countries where regulation is either poorly developed or not influenced by nurses, the profession is likely to face difficulties when trying to improve standards of education and practice and to gain greater control over its destiny. On the other hand, a regulatory body on which nurses have a strong role and that has the authority of the state to carry out its duties can become a powerful positive force. In countries where licensure is a feature of regulation and the regulatory body is funded either in whole or in part by nurses, the profession is usually strongly organized and directs its own affairs. In other countries, the development of an effective regulatory system can be instrumental in nurses gaining greater control over their profession.

Requirements for a registration system

The limitations of a registration system should be recognized. In a world with an infinite need for information, however, any system that yields information useful in decision-making and planning in the health services deserves attention and development. For example, workforce planning in health care must be based on reliable information, which regulatory systems for nursing can help to provide. To do so, such systems ideally need:

- a modern computer system;

- computer programs based on identified policies, that ensure that all relevant information is recorded and can be collated, queried and retrieved by the system;

- authority to require the registration of all students who pass the examination of a nursing education programme;

- a licensure or "effective registration" system to ensure that nurses maintain regular contact with the regulatory body and that the register is kept up to date; and

- an "information capture" exercise (retrospective record) to enable the system to obtain information from people registered before its introduction and thus to make the records as comprehensive as possible.

Systems and programs will only be effective and valuable if the policies on which they are based clearly specify their purpose and the use that will be made of the information collected. Planning such a system must take account of the financial resources and skills needed both to establish and to maintain the system.

Areas for information collection

The basic information to be recorded about each registered nurse should include: name, address, sex, age, education and dates of examinations and/or registration. The examples that follow are not exhaustive but indicate the potential of a registration system that uses a form of licensure.

Name and address. Since women predominate in the profession, a large number of nurses change their surnames as a result of marriage. Addresses also change. A system that maintains a record of names and addresses allows the computer or other system to identify registered nurses by geographical area, using postal addresses. Coupled with a licensure system that records not only the registered nurses who hold a current licence but also those who may have ceased to practise for family or other reasons, such a registration system creates the opportunity for recruitment.

As recruitment patterns change and demographic trends influence the employment market, nurses who are no longer practising become an increasingly important potential resource for the health services. The register can become a recruitment tool by encouraging nurses to return to the profession (while protecting personal information held by the regulatory body), and indicate how many professional nurses are practising and how many have ceased.

Sex and age. Even though most nurses are female, a record that shows changing patterns in recruitment by sex can be of value. In some countries, for example, initiatives have been taken to recruit more men. If linked with the licensure system, the register can show trends in the recruitment and retention of female and male recruits.

Age is a particularly important factor. The initial entry shows the nurse's age at the time of registration and the licensure system shows nurses who have retired (and thus do not require a licence). Families or others report deaths to the regulatory body in response to a licence reminder or other regular contact.

When linked with the record of education and qualifications, the register can provide an age profile of the profession. This is critically important to human resource planning. Searching the register for people of a particular age and with particular qualifications makes it possible to predict requirements for skilled nurses. For example, if health policy requires development in community or primary health services and the register shows the majority of trained community nurses to be near the age of retirement, urgent action is needed.

A registration system that also includes an index of the nursing students in education programmes will allow human resource planning to begin at an earlier stage. For example, information on population trends that predict an increase in the birth rate will require action to ensure that an adequate level of midwifery skill is available. A link between the number of student midwives, the projected birth rate and the age profile of practising midwives will provide a basis for health managers to adjust the number of places for midwifery students, increase recruitment and take other appropriate steps.

Education and qualifications. The registration system may record initial registration following a programme of education (called basic, preregistration or qualifying education) and any subsequent programmes of specialist education (called postbasic, post-registration or post-qualification education). Regular contact through the licensure system keeps this record up to date, thus providing a profile of the education and the skills of the nurses. As mentioned, a system programmed to link types of information can paint a picture, for example, of the skills and ages of nurses in a particular geographical area.

Other information and applications. Provided the framework for a registration system exists and a computer or other system is available to support it, other information can be used and correlations made according to need. For example, nurses renewing their licences may be asked to state the area of nursing in which they intend to practise in the following year. This further refinement yields even more precise information about changes in and the intentions of the professional population.

Conclusion

A live registration system can be used to construct a unique professional profile of individual registered nurses and of the profession as a whole, and forms an important part of a regulatory system for nursing. Investment in the development of a regulatory system is an important strategy in the search to create a well informed, responsible profession capable of providing appropriate and effective nursing services when and where they are needed.

4

Reorienting nursing education

The Need for Change

Changing nursing practice, particularly the fundamental change that the health for all movement requires of the nursing profession, requires changing nursing education in an equally fundamental, proactive way. Each country's new nurses need a different way of thinking, a different approach to their professional work and an expanded role.

Making primary health care the core of the curriculum will prepare the nurse of the future for a role that includes not only hospital nursing, with its central focus on disease and cure, but also community nursing. The curriculum should emphasize assisting and enabling people to meet their own health needs, fostering the maintenance and promotion of health, and providing health education, along with care in the community. The complexity and implications of the changes required to reorient nursing curricula in this direction should not be underestimated. Nurse teachers, clinical nurses and nurse managers will have to work together to pursue the aims of this exciting and challenging exercise *(22)*:

> Educators alone cannot bring about the needed change in schools of nursing or in any educational system. It is also necessary to involve, for example, ministries of health, the legislative or regulatory bodies that set the rules and regulations for nursing education, health professionals and community health consumers. Most important, it is essential that the nursing profession be committed to the need for change in nursing education and practice, and that nurses themselves become more actively involved in the change process.

Focusing on health does not mean neglecting the study of disease and the care of ill people. It does, however, mean striking a balance in the

61

education and preparation of nurses, and focusing on the dynamic, multidimensional concept of health that encompasses individuals and families and their communities.

Nurses also need to understand the beliefs and values of the people they serve, and to recognize that people differ in their values for health and health behaviour. People's knowledge and understanding of health become integral parts of each individual and community belief system. The traditional reductionist view labels patients with particular diseases or disabilities and as passive and powerless recipients of health care. This must be replaced by a more balanced view. Comprehensive care that takes account of patients' views, culture and health beliefs, and in which their positions as members of their families, groups and communities is also significant, must become the norm. People must have relevant information to be able to participate in and to influence their care.

Planning the Change

Change equals challenge. What better challenge could nurses tackle than working together to create, implement and evaluate a new curriculum for nursing education? Change takes time. The curriculum will not be changed overnight, but a realistic assessment of the incremental nature of many of the detailed changes, and the setting of short and longer term goals, will do much to sustain nurses' efforts. Change meets opposition; it is important not to underestimate the difficulties.

The decision to reorient the basic nursing curriculum to focus on primary health care is usually made at the highest level of government. The intended starting date and the phasing-in time may also be decided at that level, along with major resource issues. A committee should be set up at this national or federal level, with members representing nursing practice, management, education and research and, when appropriate, representatives of others with an important stake in the work, such as ministries, nursing associations, trade unions and other professional groups.

It may be necessary to create a special committee at an intermediate (perhaps regional) level to link the policy-makers and the people who will plan the curricula in schools or departments of nursing. This committee should include a representative range of nurses. While not directly involved in curriculum planning, it could be responsible for policy implementation, ensuring that resources are channelled appropriately.

The choice of level will depend on the circumstances in each Member State, including the degree of centralization of the nursing education system, and the motivation and expertise available. The ideal combination is a national or regional task force working closely with pioneering schools in which the changes will be introduced, and national and local planning groups with overlapping membership.

Direct responsibility for planning and implementing the new curriculum should rest with a planning group created at the local level, in each school or department of nursing. The groups should include nurse teachers, practising nurses and nurse researchers and managers who represent both hospital and community nursing. If more than one type of nursing education is the norm in the country (if there are both degree and diploma programmes, for example), then teachers representing both programmes should participate. The inclusion of representatives from the clinical and management parts of the health service is essential.

Any rules and regulations governing the nursing profession must be borne in mind, including international directives or standards such as those of the Council of Europe *(23)* and the European Community *(24)*. Compliance with the minimum requirements stated in the European Community directives is a necessary prerequisite to the free movement of professional nurses within the Community: the minimum full-time study period must comprise a three-year course or 4600 hours of theoretical and practical instruction. The Council of Europe agreement recommends that the theoretical component be not less than one third and the practice component not less than half of the total programme.

Action: stage 1

The following steps are recommended to each curriculum planning group, whether at the national or local level. Each planning group should assess what needs to be changed in the curriculum, identify goals and objectives, plan strategies and tactics to ensure that the reoriented curriculum becomes a reality, implement the change with colleagues over an agreed period and, finally, decide on the evaluation of the change. As mentioned, communication with the people who support the change at more senior policy-making levels is vital. The group should:

(a) read through and discuss the Declaration of Alma-Ata *(2)* and the 38 regional targets for health for all *(25)*;

(b) consider their implications for the health service of the country and in particular for the basic nursing education curriculum;

(c) debate the concept of health;

(d) discuss the changing role of the nurse;

(e) identify the various groups that will be affected by or should be involved in changing the curriculum;

(f) conduct a preliminary analysis of the strengths and weaknesses of the present nursing curriculum;

(g) outline the major changes likely to be necessary when the new curriculum is designed and implemented;

(h) consider the possible future curriculum changes under these three headings *(26)*: a stable condition and the present reality, moderate changes in the near future or transformation later; and

(i) record decisions and key areas for action on all these issues, and identify the group member responsible for taking each action.

Educational Outcomes or Competences

The essential first step in designing a reoriented curriculum is to decide on the competences to be expected of the nurse. What should be the outcomes of the new programme? These will be comprehensive and are best expressed in broad terms. Detail should be added at the later stage of planning the content of the curriculum.

A number of lists of competences or outcomes now exist. The participants at a WHO consultation on curriculum development *(27)* agreed that education must enable the nurse:

(a) to select information to enable her to assess, plan, deliver and evaluate nursing care for individuals, families, groups or communities;

(b) to apply pertinent research to nursing practice;

(c) to apply a problem-solving approach to care, taking particular measures as appropriate;

(d) to contribute to the organization and deployment of care;

(e) to participate in the teaching, monitoring and supervision of others;

(f) to be accountable for the care she gives;

(g) to contribute effectively to the multidisciplinary team;

(h) to cooperate with people and agencies in a variety of settings for the benefit of individuals, families and communities;

(i) to understand the importance of the ethics of health care and of the nursing profession and their influence on nurses' professional practice;

(j) to apply current legislation governing health care;

(k) to respond to changing influences governing health care; and

(l) to assess the political and policy issues surrounding and influencing nursing practice.

McMurray *(28)* cites other competences for the community health nurse that may stimulate debate. These are:

basic nursing skills; basic knowledge of wellness and illness; clear understanding of the focus of public health; ability to apply the nursing process – to assess, plan, implement and evaluate care for clients and client groups; documentation and communication skills; the ability to interpret public health and community health nursing to consumers, other health professionals, and the community; ability to plan time and set priorities for workloads; ability to teach and counsel; ability to solve problems, make decisions, and understand and implement change; knowledge of community resources and how to use them; understanding of the relationship of finances to service delivery; ability to work with others.

Competences raise certain key issues that must be dealt with at the policy-making level. The decisions made must then be implemented in the design of the reoriented curriculum. These key issues include recruitment, the availability of entrants with sufficient academic qualifications to tackle the new programme, and levels of preparation and articulation between these levels, not only for current and future students but also for the qualified workforce.

Recruitment, entry qualifications and age

If the competences quoted above or similar ones are to be attained, they will require the recruitment of a well educated student. As mentioned earlier, the participants at the European Conference on Nursing recommended that students accepted for nursing training should have had the general education required for entry into university (Annex 1). In 1989, the Commission of the European Communities recommended that nurses' preparation in the twenty-first century should be at university level *(29)*. Not every country may be able immediately to have student nurses with a minimum of 12 years of school education before entry to the profession; this may be a long-term goal. An early aim, however, should be to ensure that the minimum age of entry is 17 years.

The level of the award

The award gained on qualification should not only permit formal registration as a nurse, but also have academic credit valued at or above the level of diploma. In many countries, nursing education has developed alongside rather than as an integral part of the higher education system; thus, academic accreditation may require initial negotiation at the national policy-making level.

Many countries have two levels of preparation, with a majority of nurses achieving a diploma and a smaller proportion graduating with a degree in nursing. The diploma, as well as the degree, should have academic recognition that will permit nurses to enter advanced degree-level preparation later should they so wish. The academic credit points should be able to be used within the credit accumulation and transfer scheme being developed throughout Europe *(30)*.

Minimum period of study

A a long-term goal, the minimum period of full-time study must not be less than three years. This should be inclusive of holidays, but exclusive of sickness or absence for any other reason. As noted previously, the programme must contain not less than 4600 hours of learning to comply with a European Community directive *(24)*.

Staffing implications

So that student nurses may study and gain experience, it is assumed that they will not be part of the health service workforce during their basic preparation, that is, they will be supernumerary. In some countries this is already the case; where it is not, this principle has major staffing implications that must be handled within the overall policies on nursing. Experience in one Member State has shown that this transition may be less disruptive than expected.

Action: stage 2

In this stage of the review and reorientation of the curriculum, the planning group should:

(a) in consultation with key members of the profession and national policy-makers, prepare the list of outcomes or competences that nurses must attain on completion of their basic education within the reoriented curriculum;

(b) learn about the national demographic trends and projections for the next 30–40 years, particularly in relation to the group aged 15–25 years;

(c) with experts in human resource development, discuss trends in and projections for other professions;

(d) obtain national forecasts of the future needs for health professionals, including the categories and mixes of staff likely to be required;

(e) discuss with nurses at policy-making levels the country's position on the key issues of recruitment, educational qualifications

and age on entry to nursing education, academic levels of preparation, articulation between levels and eligibility for credit transfer across the European Region; and

(f) set requirements for these as the basis of the reoriented curriculum.

The Reoriented Curriculum

The major subjects in the reoriented curriculum will be nursing and health. Other subjects – such as life sciences, epidemiology, psychology, sociology, research appreciation and application, communication, ethics and political awareness – are also important. Nursing must nevertheless carry the greatest weight and must be closely integrated with the study of health.

The nature of nursing requires that nurses gain the relevant knowledge, skills and attitudes in the classroom and clinical practice, whether in a hospital or the community. Just as it is essential to define the competences expected of nurses qualifying from the reoriented curriculum, it is also of fundamental importance to agree on the nature of nursing. The process of education and training will inevitably transmit values and beliefs to students and to the qualified workforce.

The planning group would be well advised to widen its discussions by involving people who have significant contact with students and those who may influence the proposed learning environment. This should help to avoid conflict later. Crucial issues include:

- the nature of nursing and therefore the value placed on different subjects in the course and how they are taught and assessed;

- what constitutes nursing knowledge – whether it stems from a particular discipline and is transmitted through the nursing process and models of nursing, or is merely an amalgam from a number of different disciplines; and

- how best to foster the development of the nurse in the classroom and in the practice setting.

No one has yet been able to create a universally acceptable philosophy of nursing. That may not matter, however, because part of the importance of the attempt to do so is that the people involved discuss their essential beliefs (about the individual, society, health and nursing) and plan how to share these with others.

In writing a philosophy, the planning group may choose to adopt or adapt the WHO statement on the mission of nursing (see Chapter 1). The group should not prepare a lengthy document, but use everyday language and plan with idealism tempered with realism. The philosophy of nursing should contain key concepts; people's beliefs about these will determine the knowledge required for nursing practice. Everyone involved in the nursing programme, whether as student, teacher, practising nurse or manager, must be clear about the fundamental values and beliefs that will underpin the reoriented curriculum.

A systematic approach to nursing

Nurses must adopt a more comprehensive approach to care, delivered on a systematic basis and guided by a specific conceptual approach. The curriculum should provide for the teaching of this systematic approach, which is frequently called the nursing process, and is enhanced by the use of a theoretical framework or nursing model that represents the totality of nursing viewed from a particular theoretical perspective. Using a nursing model enables the identification of the essential components of comprehensive care; the planning group should consider using this tool.

The number of nursing models is large and still growing. No one model is equally applicable to all the circumstances in which nursing care is given, but that devised by Roper et al. *(31)* and based on a earlier model created by Henderson in 1960 *(32)* may be a useful start. It has been widely accepted and can be used in both community and hospital. It provides a framework for examining the health maintaining and health promoting aspects of the lifestyles of individuals and groups in the following activities of living:

- maintaining a safe environment
- communicating
- breathing
- eating and drinking

- eliminating
- personal cleansing and dressing
- controlling body temperature
- mobilizing
- working and playing
- expressing sexuality
- sleeping
- dying.

This provides a clear and simple framework within which to identify and analyse a person's actual and potential health problems, and thus to develop specific topics in the curriculum. On communicating, for example, nursing education might include the examination of: elements of communication, barriers and aids to communication, interactive skills, making verbal and written reports, and issues of confidentiality.

This model offers a person-centred approach. It views nursing as helping people to prevent, alleviate, solve or cope with problems related to daily living. It acknowledges the influence of biological, psychological, sociocultural, environmental and political factors on the person's ability to perform the activities of living. Finally, it recognizes that nurses can and do provide care for people throughout their life span, from conception to death, and at any point on a continuum from health to ill health, from dependence to independence. Their aim is to enable people to realize maximum potential and as much independence as possible.

The reoriented curriculum emphasizes the community. As the curriculum content and learning experiences are organized, the planning group should monitor them regularly, to ensure that they are consistent with the primary health care approach. Table 1 gives a comparison of traditional and community health orientations to nursing.

Action: stage 3

In this stage of the review and reorientation of the curriculum, the planning group should:

(a) clarify the values that underpin the current curriculum and thus the practice of nursing;

(b) agree on the key concepts to be developed in the reoriented educational programme;

(c) following consultation, agree on the philosophy of the reoriented curriculum;

(d) consider to what extent the medical model dominates the present curriculum, and what changes would be required to give a central role to caring;

(e) discuss the location of the present curriculum on the continuum between the traditional approach and a community health orientation;

(f) discuss the implications of adopting a systematic approach to nursing using a nursing model; and

(g) before any detailed consideration of the content of the curriculum, work through and agree on the implementation in the reoriented curriculum of a nursing model that is congruent with the central role of nursing and that uses a systematic approach to care.

The Curriculum Content

The core concepts of the individual (man, woman or child), the social and physical environments, health and nursing are the focus of all subjects in the curriculum. The student of nursing should begin by studying health and the healthy person, the healthy environment and the healthy community, before proceeding to the study of deviations from optimum health. Most students begin with an image of nursing that focuses on the hospital and is rather dramatic. The planning group must be prepared to defend the primary health care focus of the reoriented curriculum as the most appropriate to the country's needs, as identified on the basis of demographic, epidemiological and social data. Thus, the emphasis on some subjects may vary between countries, areas within a country or urban, suburban and rural districts.

Nursing is both a science and an art. It is also based on research. While much of the relevant theoretical knowledge will be taught and learned in the classroom, the application of that knowledge must be taught and learned in contact with people in the primary health care or hospital setting. If nurses are to function effectively, their education must be

Table 1. Comparison of traditional and community health orientation to nursing practice – educational focus

Curriculum characteristics	Traditional nursing	Community-oriented focus
Primary focus	Sick individual (patterned on the curative model)	Community health (patterned on demographic, socioeconomic and environmental health model for self-reliance in health)
Target population	Sick and disabled seeking health care	Total population, especially the underserved and high-risk groups
Primary settings for learning	Hospitals, other institutions, the home	Wherever people are
Nursing role	Specialized and interdependent within the health sector	Broad, independent and interdependent in the health and health-related sectors
Nursing concerns	Conditions requiring hospitalization	Promoting health, preventing disease/disability, rehabilitation, care and support Prevailing health problems and needs of the community
Nursing practice	Nursing care of individuals Patient/family participation in care Some follow-up of patients through hospital outpatient department	Primary health care approach Enabling community/family/client/patient involvement in care Identification and follow-up of vulnerable groups, with health team approach to care
Problem-solving process	Assessment of individual and family needs and resources Intervention through individual and family	Transfer of knowledge and skill to enable community/group/family/individual to meet needs Enabling self-determination by community/group/family/individual

Table 1. *(contd)*

Curriculum characteristics	Traditional nursing	Community-oriented focus
Objectives of practice		
Prevention	Focus on secondary/tertiary prevention	Focus on primary prevention
Therapy	Patient well enough to be discharged	Improved health and nutritional status of patient, family and community, self-care, self-reliance
Health care delivery system	Institutional and individualized care of patients	Primary health care for all, involvement of other sectors influencing health, health team approach
Evaluation of nursing practice	Number of patients discharged from care by diagnostic category	Percentage of population covered, consumer satisfaction, quality assurance
	Frequency and intensity of patient contact	Rates of change in health status of high-risk groups/community
		Rates of response in "treated" groups, i.e., immunization, therapy, average length of hospitalization, self-care ability, and changes in health behaviour and lifestyles. Reduction in environmental health hazards

Source: A guide to curriculum review for basic nursing education (22).

73

grounded in and derived from practice. Progress through the curriculum could demonstrate the development of knowledge and skills of increasing complexity. Subjects must be interrelated and their relevance to practice reinforced. Two important elements of the curriculum, as in education for all practice-based disciplines, are the integration of theory and practice, and experiential learning. In preparing to design the details of the curriculum, the group may find it helpful to use a form such as the one given in Fig. 4 in relation to each syllabus element.

As the major focus of the curriculum, the study of the theory and practice of nursing should carry the most weight – reflected in the allocation of a greater number of curriculum hours. Health promotion and health education are closely integrated with nursing and they should occupy more curriculum hours than other supporting subjects.

Other important subjects to be covered in the curriculum include:

- human development and the relationship of health to the social environment;
- the social and behavioural sciences;
- communication skills;
- organizational structures and processes; and
- professional, ethical and moral issues in nursing.

The curriculum could address many topics under each of these headings; some lists are given in the box at the end of this chapter.

The programme should include a systematic approach to nursing care in which the nurse:

- applies an appropriate model of nursing;
- identifies needs or problems in cooperation with clients and selects additional information from other sources;
- sets achievable short- and long-term goals;
- plans acute intervention, using practical and technical skills;
- implements care and evaluates progress towards agreed objectives;
- promotes independence and self-care;
- maintains a safe environment;

- contributes as a team member in programmes of care, supervision and rehabilitation with other professional groups; and
- develops an inquiring approach to nursing practice, taking account of research.

Interdisciplinary modules should be included in the later years of the course, when the students know and feel confident about their roles. Modules on the roles of other health workers should be included to emphasize the importance of interprofessional cooperation.

Action: stage 4

In this stage of the review and reorientation of the curriculum, the planning group should:

(a) consider the subjects included in the curriculum, especially in relation to demographic, epidemiological and social data, the new elements on primary health care, and the clinical learning that will be available in institutions and the community (this should be done in close consultation with colleagues at all levels of the health care system);

(b) set up specialist groups of teachers who, in consultation with colleagues in practice and management, will plan the detailed content of the community health and nursing syllabuses;

(c) set up similar specialist groups to plan the detailed content of the syllabuses for the supporting disciplines;

(d) make arrangements to ensure liaison between everyone involved; and

(e) review and finalize the total subject content to ensure harmony with the governing philosophy and balance within the overall curriculum.

The complete syllabuses will contain the learning objectives, subject content and reading lists, and information on the teaching and learning strategies and the methods of assessment to be used.

Fig. 4. Integration of theory and practice in nursing education

This could be appropriate under the general heading of health promotion and health education.
Please check (x) the *appropriate* column(s) for each *individual term* and indicate the year(s) taught and number of hours for each section and sub-section of the syllabus.

Concepts of health and wellness: some possible content	Objectives	Year(s) taught	Lecture	Role playing/ simulation	Self-instruction/ process recordings	Demonstration/ observation	Supervised clinical practice	Evaluation of student learning
1. Human relationships and the helping process								
(a) self-awareness								
(b) self-values								
(c) self-esteem/identity								
(d) self-motivation								
(e) self-care								
(f) reaction to loss								
(g) assertiveness/leadership								
(h) interpersonal relationships								
2. Communication								
(a) nonverbal/observation								
(b) verbal/listening								
(c) interviewing								
(d) counselling								
(e) teaching/health education								
(f) empathic caring								
(g) family interaction								

Fig. 4. (contd)

Concepts of health and wellness: some possible content	Objectives	Year(s) taught	Lecture	Role playing/ simulation	Self-instruction/ process recordings	Demonstration/ observation	Supervised clinical practice	Evaluation of student learning
3. Human psychology and health behaviour								
(a) human needs								
(b) attitudes/perceptions								
(c) values, beliefs								
(d) cultural practices								
(e) health behaviour								
(f) learning and motivation								
(g) reaction to crisis								
4. Psychosocial development								
(a) infant stimulation								
(b) preschool development								
(c) youth — self-esteem/social competence								
(d) maternal and family development								
(e) family planning/human sexuality								
(f) team or group work								
(g) work skills and satisfaction								
(h) creativity and generativity of aging								

Source: Integration of a model health component in general nursing education (33).

Integration of Theory and Practice

The planning group must address the following issues in order to encourage the integration of theory and practice.

Curriculum structure

The structure or sequencing of the curriculum should, as far as possible, juxtapose theoretical teaching with relevant practice. A curriculum designed in modules will help: a form of sandwich, in which theory is followed by relevant practice and then by a period of consolidation to encourage reflection.

Curriculum process

Both teaching and learning strategies can help or hinder the integration of theory and practice. Many students have difficulty in transferring classroom learning to clinical practice and, at least in the early stages, in transferring learning from their work experience in one setting to another. This is partly a result of teaching strategies that do not make it clear that transfer is possible and expected. All students tend to search for facts, the right or wrong way to do something, the one right answer, the rules to follow. Their teachers know that students must learn to apply their theoretical knowledge in different ways.

Students should be taught to expect apparent ambiguities, made aware of the contextual and relative nature of knowledge, and supported and supervised by skilled nurse teachers when they are finding this out. Without support and supervision, they may learn to discount the teaching and learning done in the school. They may reject the theoretical underpinning that is essential to the advancement of nursing, and become disillusioned in a fruitless search for one right way to deliver care. They may never learn to become active learners and reflective practitioners who can cope with the challenge of change.

Teaching practice-based nursing

In the reoriented curriculum, many practice placements will be in the primary health care setting, in stark contrast to the traditional curriculum.

The WHO consultation on curriculum development *(27)* defined community-based education as "a means of achieving educational relevance to community needs", and included in a list of community-based learning activities:

- assignment to a family whose health care is observed over a period of time;

- work in an urban, suburban or rural community to gain an understanding of the relationship of the health sector to other sectors engaged in community development, and of the social system, including the dominance of some groups over others;

- participation in a community survey, diagnosis and action plan, or in a programme on immunization, health education, nutrition or child care, for example; and

- supervised work at a primary care facility.

The reoriented curriculum must include placements in primary, secondary and tertiary health care settings, and provide opportunities for nurses to practise all aspects of their role. The students should learn in an environment that closely resembles that in which they will work on completion of their basic nurse education. Community-based education is therefore not an end in itself, but a means of ensuring that health personnel are responsive to the health needs of the people.

In designing the elements of the curriculum related to the community, the planning group may find a WHO report helpful *(34)*. To be effective, the programme must fulfil certain conditions and conform to certain guiding principles. The students' activities should relate to planned educational goals and objectives, and students and teachers must have a clear understanding of the purpose and the expected results. The activities should be introduced very early in the educational experience and continue throughout the programme. They must be viewed not as peripheral or casual experiences but as a standard, integral and continuing part of the educational process. The students' work during training must be real work, related to their educational needs, and form part of the requirements for obtaining a degree. Further, the objectives of a community-based educational programme differ markedly from those of traditional field work. The programme must clearly benefit both the student and the community, which implies that the community must be actively involved. In addition, the teachers of nursing in the practice areas must be experts, whether they are nurse teachers or practitioners.

Practising nurses also have a crucial contribution to make in supervising, teaching and acting as role models for the students. It is practising nurses who create the climate for learning. Community and clinical areas that receive students on placement will normally have been approved by the regulatory body and/or the educational institution offering the programme; they will be able to offer appropriate experience and have enough staff for adequate supervision. Preferably, each placement area should have an organized teaching programme for the students it receives.

The progression from supervised hands-on experience to independent practice should be gradual. Whether given certain tasks or the responsibility for total patient care, students should always be encouraged to see their work in context. Before and after the experience, tutorials and small group discussions, case conferences (some of which may be able to include the client) and exercises for discussion in the tutorials (such as the keeping of a learning diary and notes of critical incidents) can all help students to reflect on and learn from their actions.

The planning group should note the many implications of such changes for nurse teachers and for the qualified workforce. A later section of this chapter examines the preparation of people who will teach and supervise students in the reoriented curriculum.

Action: stage 5

In this stage of the review and reorientation of the curriculum, the planning group should:

(a)   discuss the different types of knowledge relevant to the study of nursing, and decide where and how they will be transmitted within the reoriented curriculum;

(b)   discuss how theory and practice are integrated in the present curriculum, and debate how they will be integrated in the structure, timetable and process of the new curriculum;

(c) discuss and agree with colleagues in the community on the provision of a suitable range of placements for community-based nurse education, while not neglecting the need to continue the use of suitable placements in secondary and tertiary care settings;

(d) discuss the role of practising nurses in the transmission to students of the values, knowledge and skills of nursing in the reoriented curriculum, and the preparation they might require to act as mentors; and

(e) create an integrated curriculum based on theory and practice.

Teaching and Learning Strategies

Inevitably, the reoriented curriculum will require not only new content but also new teaching strategies, and will alter the way in which the students learn.

In essence, the difference between the traditional and the progressive approaches to nursing preparation lies in the difference between education and training, and between educating adults and educating children. The art and science of helping adults learn is based on the following assumptions: that an adult's self-concept moves from that of a dependent personality towards that of a self-directing human being; that an adult accumulates a growing reservoir of experience that becomes an increasing resource for learning; that an adult's readiness to learn increasingly focuses on the tasks inherent in her social (and professional) roles; and that an adult's time perspective changes from the postponed application of knowledge to immediacy of application, and accordingly an adult shifts from a concern with subject matter to a concern to use knowledge to solve challenges and problems in their context.

The end of the transition from student entrant to competent qualified nurse cannot be precisely defined, so the teaching and learning strategies adopted in the reoriented curriculum must maximize the individual's potential to develop the broad competences outlined previously. The student nurse must be educated and trained, but the historical emphasis on training must now shift to education. The student nurse must of course be trained in many specific types of behaviour, such as learning to calculate drug dosages, to complete a fluid balance chart, to handle forceps and to carry out aseptic techniques. The application of these techniques, however, will involve very different behaviour, too complex to specify precisely beforehand, because it will depend on the context in which the nursing is carried out. To achieve this, nurses need more than training: they also need education.

The major focus, therefore, is to assist adults to learn how to learn: to become self-directed learners. This has implications for the teacher. The relationship between teacher and student changes and the student's dependence on the teacher decreases – not an easy shift for teachers used to a rather authoritarian, controlled and didactic approach to teaching. The emphasis of the teaching and learning process shifts from the teacher to the student. As student and teacher become used to the new approach, there is more negotiation between them on what and how the student will learn. The teacher becomes a facilitator of learning, someone who supports the student's quest for knowledge. This facilitator role is particularly relevant when the knowledge to be taught is contextual and relative, as in nursing.

A successful move from traditional to progressive teaching and learning will be gradual and planned. It is also important to take account of the effect of such a change on the qualified nurses who will receive these students in the clinical areas. Fig. 5 shows the progression from teacher-centred to student-centred teaching and learning strategies.

Fig. 5 includes both teaching and assessment methods. In addition to lectures, most of which should encourage questioning and discussion, the strategies include demonstrations, tutorials, seminars (many of which should be led by the students), skills analysis and demonstrations, computer-assisted learning, role playing, practice-based experiential learning and self-directed learning. Many of these require dividing the class into small groups, which has resource implications in terms of teachers' numbers and time, as well as implications for how students' learning is assessed.

The use of small group teaching and self-directed learning also has resource implications for library accommodation, the provision of books and journals, and the need for seminar and study rooms. The reoriented curriculum will require students to spend time in the library. No longer will they only listen passively to the teacher as the fount of all knowledge: they must read, question, reflect on and critically analyse their new knowledge, and then apply it to their practice.

The change to the progressive approach to education also has major implications for practising nurses and nurse managers, who will be faced with a thinking, questioning student. How they deal with the new breed of nurse is crucial, and the planning group must consider how to prepare them for the change and obtain their support.

Fig. 5. Progression from teacher-centred to student-centred teaching and learning strategies

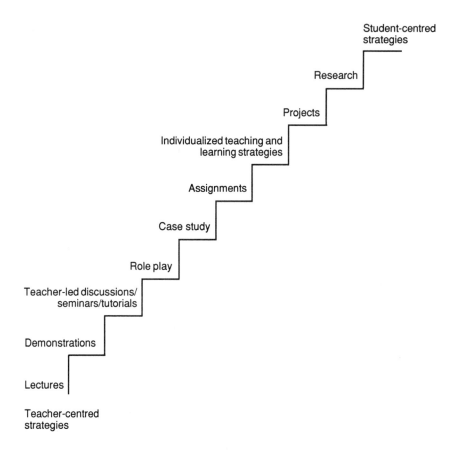

Source: Managing change in nursing education. Pack 1 (35).

Action: stage 6

In this stage of the review and reorientation of the curriculum, the members of the planning group should:

(a)   consider the present position of their school's curriculum on a scale ranging from the education of children to that of adults;

(b)   consider the time required and other implications of emphasizing adult teaching and learning strategies in the curriculum;

(c)   decide and agree on the appropriate teaching and learning strategies for the various subjects; and

(d)   liaise with colleagues to arrange appropriate preparation for all the teachers involved and the qualified nurses who will supervise the students in their placement experiences.

Assessment

The challenge for curriculum planners in nursing is to choose forms of assessment that will predict as exactly as possible the students' fitness to practise and how they might approach their practice in years to come (34):

> How the students' performance is to be evaluated must be decided at an early stage, since it will influence how other aspects of the programme are planned. The assessment of competence in applying the concept of primary health care must be a requirement for certification, not only to protect the community from the ministration of incompetent health personnel but also to ensure that the students do not disregard the primary health care orientation of the curriculum. Assessment instruments must therefore be constructed to measure how the students perform each of the professional tasks, including those for which competence can be acquired through community-based learning activities.

An assessment schedule is an integral part of any curriculum, and it is most important that this be designed at the same time as the curriculum is developed. The assessment strategies should be congruent with the philosophy, aims, teaching strategies and intended outcomes of the curriculum. For example, it is useless to adopt adult teaching and learning strategies that require students to reflect on practice and think creatively in solving health care problems in various settings, and then assess their performance with examinations that require only the regurgitation of context-free, factual knowledge and test only memorization skills. Instead, assessments should lead the students to think and use their problem-solving skills.

Many countries try to achieve a national standard by means of a national system of examinations, centrally controlled and administered. In other countries the system of examinations is devolved to institutions that must be approved by the higher education authorities and the professional regulatory body.

Education for a practice-based profession such as nursing prepares students to undertake a responsible role that is defined by law in most countries, and thus has an obligation to produce a safe and competent practitioner. Assessment is vital to the monitoring and maintenance of standards. Examinations and assessments also provide feedback to teachers on their effectiveness and to students on their progress. Valid assessment procedures can highlight students' strengths and weaknesses and enable them to seek appropriate help from their teachers or from expert practitioners of nursing. In giving feedback, teachers should always try to influence the behaviour of the students in a positive way.

A "formative assessment" provides continued feedback to students, and, by definition, does not usually count towards what is often the terminal or final assessment or examination, that is, the "summative assessment". The results of summative assessments are traditionally linked to a mark or grade. Ranking students' standing relative to other students by means of marks is called norm-referenced assessment. In nursing it seems more important to establish what students can or cannot do by criterion-referenced assessment.

Knowledge assessment

Three forms of knowledge need to be assessed (Fig. 6).

The written examination of students' achievements in the cognitive domain has traditionally predominated. This is still important, but research findings challenge the ability of written tests to predict students'

Fig. 6. Forms of knowledge to be assessed

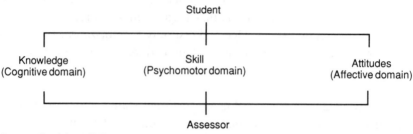

Student

| Knowledge (Cognitive domain) | Skill (Psychomotor domain) | Attitudes (Affective domain) |

Assessor

Source: Bradshaw *(36).*

success in the actual practice of nursing. For various reasons, therefore, the emphasis of examinations and assessments has gradually changed. All countries and schools of nursing are likely to be at different stages; the planning group should determine the stage of its curriculum, and consider the following current range of possibilities for assessment.

First, a written examination tests mainly theoretical knowledge, its basis in research (when relevant) and its application to practice. Examples are:

- the traditional "unseen" examination paper, using either multiple-choice items or questions that require short answers or longer essays;

- a "seen" examination, whose questions are issued to the students some time before the examination; and

- an open-book examination, in which students have usually been given the questions in advance and are permitted to take appropriate texts into the examination room.

The latter two, by allowing time for preparation, are intended to probe in more depth the students' abilities to attain higher educational objectives such as analysis, synthesis and critical thinking.

Course work provides a second opportunity for assessment. Examples are:

- essays of various lengths, in which the findings of research and theoretical concepts from nursing and the supporting disciplines are expected to be integrated and applied to practice;

86

- laboratory reports in both biological and behavioural sciences;

- projects, which may include pictorial or audiovisual material prepared for display, or seminar papers for oral presentation and subsequent submission of the written paper;

- nursing care studies, which emphasize the application of theory to practice; and

- a dissertation (usually required only in a degree programme), that is, an in-depth examination of an area of nursing of particular interest to the student (it should be research-based and usually at least 5000 words long).

The use of marking keys constructed by the teacher who sets the question or assignment improves the reliability of the marking.

The planning group, along with colleagues involved in similar groups across the country, should consider the issue of quality control and the maintenance of standards. A number of countries use a system of external examining, requiring that examination and course work assignments be checked by one or more external examiners before being given to the students; the examiners subsequently see either a sample of students' papers or, in certain cases, all of them. An external examiner provides the course team with an invaluable outside opinion, ensures fairness to the students and is able to judge the standards of the course against those of others. The examiner normally has the right to alter marks or grades if considered necessary.

These forms of assessment are used in the classroom or the laboratory under invigilation, or are completed by the students in the library or in their own homes.

Clinical assessment

It is very difficult to create a clinical assessment tool that captures the reality of practice with all its complexities, unpredictability and individuality. Such a tool must be reliable, valid and capable of predicting whether the student is or will be competent to practise. In addition to having these essential qualities, the tool must also be applicable in busy clinical areas, whether in the hospital or the community, and by a number of clinical staff who are not themselves qualified teachers. It must therefore be easily understood and require relatively little time to complete.

Much of the literature has dealt with clinical assessment in hospital settings. A WHO report discussed the assessment of competence in community-based learning activities (34):

> While there are clear advantages in ensuring that performance in actual health care practice is assessed, there are also practical difficulties ... It must be said unequivocally that students will tend to pay little attention to the primary health care aspects of a curriculum unless an assessment of their competency in applying the concept is a requirement for graduation and certification.

The following are five of the available options.

The first is a check-list. In the early days of clinical assessment, the focus was on the tasks to be performed, and this focus reflected the atomistic view of nursing held at that time. The exclusive use of check-lists – in which nursing procedures such as bed-bathing or giving an injection are broken down into steps that are ticked off as the student nurse performs them – may lead to the devaluing of the context-related, individual aspects of nursing. They can be used to observe and assess total patient care, however, and can be further enhanced by the "starring" of criterion behaviour, which the student must demonstrate in order to attain a pass mark.

Check-lists are most effectively used as a formative assessment, so that any errors (of commission or omission) can be corrected before their use as a final summative assessment. The problem with check-lists is that they measure a moment in time. They are snapshots that do not necessarily predict the student's ability to maintain a satisfactory performance.

Second, a rating scale, although a form of check-list, gives a finer judgement of a student's behaviour; an example from the community setting is given in Fig. 7. The WHO report (34) from which the example is taken highlights the lack of assessment instruments and criteria for optimum performance in the multidisciplinary community setting, and the poor quality of those that are available. The results expected from the students' activities or output (health indicators) should be used as criteria

Fig. 7. Assessment of student performance

Student's name ....

Group leader ....
(staff)

Date of posting ....

Place of posting ....

1	2	3	4	5
Unsatisfactory		Satisfactory		Distinction

Please mark X next to the appropriate number below

		Mid-posting	End of posting
1.	Appearance and general behaviour	....	....
2.	Punctuality	....	....
3.	Attitude towards the community-based education and service programme	....	....
4.	Relationship to other students	....	....
5.	Relationship to people in the community	....	....
6.	Collection of data	....	....
7.	Presentation of data	....	....
8.	Interpretation of data	....	....
9.	Ability to relate findings to solving community health problems	....	....
10.	Student's critique of his/her approach to the problems	....	....
11.	Ability to suggest new approaches to the solution of problems	....	....
12.	Contribution to group discussion	....	....
13.	Performance in crisis situation	....	....
14.	Assessment of the student's written report	....	....
	Total scores	....	....

Remarks by the group leader ....

Student's comments on his (or her) own performance. (The group leader is to discuss the performance with the student concerned at mid-posting and end of posting and enter here relevant points which might come out of the discussion).

Date .... Signature of group leader ....

Source: Community-based education of health personnel (34).

for acceptable performance whenever they are within the student's control and when no external factors can influence them. When external factors can influence these results, the process (that is, the actual activities) should be assessed. WHO also advocates the training of multidisciplinary teams of teachers in the use of a variety of instruments for assessing performance, and suggests that peer review by students is an essential element.

The third option is the critical incident technique and the learning diary. To use the critical incident technique, the teachers must agree on the core behaviour or competences that students can be expected to master at specific stages of their preparation. These can be incorporated into an assessment tool that is used when the student is observed in practice. A number of measurements must be taken, and the results aggregated.

Students can keep learning diaries during each placement, so that they may assess and reflect on their practice. This will allow them to specify their learning needs and actively seek to have these met. It also encourages students to assume more responsibility for their own learning.

Clinical placement reports are the fourth option. Placement reports were previously completed only at the very end of a clinical placement and with minimal involvement of the student. This must gradually change in the reoriented curriculum. An interim, formative assessment should be made with, not on, the student at a half-way stage in each clinical placement and then again at the final stage, as a summative assessment. The student should always take part in her assessment.

The fifth option is clinical assessment profiles. The profession's endeavours to improve unsatisfactory clinical assessment and to try to capture the twin concepts of attaining and maintaining competence have led to the relatively new concept of profiling. The clinical assessment profile offers a means of recording assessment across a wide range of the student's abilities, skills, attitudes, personal qualities and achievements, as well as her knowledge of curriculum subjects. It frequently involves the student in its formation, and has a formative as well as a summative function. Because competence is contextual, separate profiles are completed during and at the close of each clinical placement in hospital and community.

90

A single item (Fig. 8) from a profile used during a student nurse's first clinical experience in hospital or community illustrates the potential to observe progression from the initial exposure to practice (level 1) to competence (level 4), in this case in relation to administering medication *(37)*. The boxes for the levels are filled with a tick or initials as each level is reached. A profile relating to a particular placement may have 20 or more such statements.

If used correctly, the profile has the potential to present a comprehensive and developing portrayal of the student's growth towards professional competence. It is the best tool currently available for clinical assessment, but is still very much under development.

Fig. 8. Student progression from initial exposure to practice (level 1) to competence (level 4)

Statement			
Administers medications accurately and safely, monitors untoward effects, reactions, therapeutic responses, toxicity and incompatibilities.			
Level 1	Level 2	Level 3	Level 4
Understands the control, storage and administration of medicines in accordance with accepted policy and can interpret a prescription sheet correctly. ☐	Can assist a registered nurse in the administration of prescribed medicines. ☐	Administers prescribed medicines under the supervision of a registered nurse. ☐	Proficiently gives medications via usual drug administration routes. Knows the actions and common side effects of frequently prescribed medications. ☐

Source: Department of Health and Nursing Studies, Glasgow Polytechnic *(37).*

Action: stage 7

In this stage of the review and reorientation of the curriculum, the planning group should:

(a) discuss the philosophy, purpose, content and methods (tools) of assessment that would be appropriate for both the theoretical and practical elements of the reoriented curriculum;

(b) explore the difficulties inherent in the assessment of competence in clinical practice;

(c) consider how students can be involved more actively in assessment;

(d) consider what preparation will be required for the teachers and the qualified nurses who will assess the students;

(e) discuss with colleagues at the policy-making level whether a system of quality control involving external examiners can be created; and

(f) design the assessment schedule for the reoriented curriculum.

Evaluation

Evaluation is about the making of value judgements based on the systematic, scientific collection and analysis of data. The strategy for evaluating the reoriented curriculum should be planned at the same time as the curriculum is developed. To ensure that the evaluation is of value, the concepts and outcomes, syllabus content, stucture, assessment schedule and examination regulations of the course must be clearly and comprehensively documented. Data will also be needed on students (their numbers, entry qualifications, progression through the course and marks or grades achieved), teaching staff (their qualifications and areas of expertise), support staff, accommodation and support facilities (such as libraries), and information technology. In short, all that goes on in the course should be open to scrutiny.

Evaluation ensures that the curriculum is regularly reviewed and developed to take account of changing health care needs. No curriculum, however good at one time, will remain good forever. As the needs for nursing care alter, so must the preparation of the people who will give that care. Curriculum evaluation is driven by the concept of relevance; its main purposes have been listed as follows *(38)*:

- to construct and interpret a reasonably clear overall view of what is happening in a learning programme, and to compare this with curriculum intentions;

- to identify relative strengths and weaknesses as a basis for further curriculum development;

- to identify changes in [students'] abilities arising from their curriculum experiences;

- to determine the effectiveness of the curriculum in preparing [students] to undertake particular functions;

- to delineate accountability of teachers and educational managers;

- to aid management decision-making about justification of resource expenditure.

Types of evaluation

Process evaluation is a continuous evaluation, undertaken while a programme (especially a new and innovative one) is in progress. It provides feedback to teachers to enable them to adjust their teaching strategy or content if necessary. It enables prompt decision-making. Product evaluation is more concerned with outcomes, and measures end products such as learning gains, pass/fail results or competences. It tends to evaluate the whole, while process evaluation looks at the parts within the whole.

Further, formative evaluation involves continuing examination of curriculum elements and the process of delivery. Summative evaluation deals with the totality of the curriculum in terms of whether stated goals or outcomes have been met and of how well the course has achieved its goals.

"Illuminative evaluation" is an all-encompassing approach whose aims are *(39)*:

to study how [the programme] operates; how it is influenced by the various school situations in which it is applied; what those directly concerned regard as its advantages and disadvantages; and how students' intellectual tasks and academic experience are most affected. It aims to discover and document what it is like to be participating in the scheme, whether as teacher or pupil.

For use in nurse education, this approach requires that account be taken of aspects of the physical, organizational and educational milieux of the school or university and of the placement areas; of the views of students, teachers, community and hospital staff; of the processes by which the curriculum is delivered; and of the traditional outcome measures such as test and examination results and clinical assessment results.

What, when and who

Evaluation should address each of the components of the curriculum and the relationships between them. The intentions, as expressed in concepts, outcomes and objectives, should be scrutinized for continuing relevance and for their expression in the day-to-day delivery of the curriculum. Additional examples of what may be evaluated include:

- the number of students admitted to the course, and details such as their entry qualifications;
- student performance and progression through the course;
- clinical placements;
- reports from external examiners;
- reports from student representatives;
- developments on the curriculum (changes introduced since the review);
- requirements for additional resources;
- types of scholarly activity currently undertaken by teaching staff, including research, and other staff and development activities that will underpin the teaching on the course; and
- any organizational matters that affect the course.

When fundamental changes are proposed, such as the reoriented curriculum, programme evaluation should be undertaken at regular intervals. Dynamic changes in community health status, in epidemiology or in preventive strategies will also increase the need for frequent curriculum evaluation.

The evaluation of a professional curriculum is a professional matter. The evaluation team should include nurse educators and their colleagues from nursing practice and management, and experts from the other disciplines that contribute to the programme. Formative, continuing evaluation, along with the responsibility for the arrangement of the summative evaluation (often called validation), should be an integral part of the procedures of the school or university responsible for the programme.

The use of evaluation results is a sensitive and important issue. A range of groups will be interested in the results, not just those directly involved in delivering the programme, but also those who will work with and employ the student on qualification. Other health care professionals will also be interested, especially as their own curricula should be evaluated in a similar way. Still others – such as the course management committees, academic validating bodies, statutory nursing bodies, and those who fund nurse education, whether government or university politicians and administrators – will have views on the expected benefits.

Inevitably, some elements of the curriculum will be found to work better than others. When a particular element is not praised, the person responsible for it may take this as a personal criticism. It is important to be aware that this can happen and, from the very beginning, to approach curriculum planning, development, delivery and evaluation as a team enterprise.

Action: stage 8

In this final stage of the review and reorientation of the curriculum, the planning group should:

(a) identify the issues to be considered when planning the evaluation of the reoriented curriculum;

(b) discuss these issues with relevant groups and decide on the extent, type and structure of the evaluation, and who should be involved in it;

(c) make an appropriate schedule for progress review and evaluation; and

(d) consider with nurses at the policy-making level how the results of the evaluation should be disseminated and then used to ensure continuing relevance of the curriculum to health needs.

Curriculum content – Lists of topics

The following lists are neither exhaustive nor prescriptive. They are offered as a guide for adaptation to local needs.

Theory and practice of nursing

Nursing knowledge and its application in practice are central to the programme and include:

- the characteristics of nursing
- the evolution of nursing knowledge, values, attitudes, concepts and ideologies
- the concept of care
- the nursing process
- models of nursing
- factors influencing the development of nursing practice
- the appreciation and application of research
- the application of the principles of nursing to different age groups and practice settings
- diagnostic investigations and relevant nursing actions
- methods of treatment and outcomes in relation to nursing responsibilities and actions related to normal functioning
- rehabilitation, pharmacology, emergency care and nursing responsibilities and activities
- alternative approaches to care.

Human development and the social environment

The nursing student should study normal human development (from conception to death) and normal living activities, including:

- normal human growth, development, structure, function and degeneration
- family patterns and dynamics
- culture, customs, traditions and their influences on health
- social relationships
- the nature, structure and causation of disorder and disability
- health and nutritional assessments
- community assessment
- disease processes related to normal structure and function, etiology, pathology, clinical features and the normal course of disease
- the identification of common diseases associated with the body systems and the senses (throughout the life span).

Health promotion and health education

Topics for study in promoting, maintaining and restoring health include:

- the primary health care approach to achieving health for all
- the WHO regional targets for health for all
- concepts of health education and health promotion (at the primary, secondary and tertiary levels of a health care system
- essentials for health in daily living
- family planning
- social, environmental, political, cultural and economic factors that affect health
- screening techniques
- individual, family and community assessments
- the maximum realization of health potential
- the promotion of independent living, self-care and self-help
- enabling and supporting individuals, families and communities
- the use of health data in identification of target or vulnerable individuals and groups
- teaching methods and techniques
- the planning and evaluation of health education programmes on preconception, pregnancy, preschool and school-age children, adolescents, young adults, older adults and elderly people
- administrative structures for health education at the country or district levels
- methods of facilitating change, informed choice and persuasion
- environmental health
- occupational health.

Social and behavioural sciences

The curriculum should include the study of human beings in their environment:

- the social and economic context
- normal psychological development
- families, groups, communities and their interdependence
- group dynamics
- sociology, including concepts of social structure and control
- ethnic and cultural differences, including the beliefs and practices of minority groups
- the influence of social policy on health and health care
- the study of social organizations and institutions, voluntary organizations, and national and international health organizations and their responsibilities
- the activities of daily living
- the interrelationship of psychological processes and physical function
- sociological perspectives of health and illness.

Communication skills

Topics should include:

- self-awareness and sensitivity to others
- verbal and nonverbal communication
- the development of communication skills
- communication with different cultural and ethnic groups, impaired or disabled people, and colleagues (individually and as team members)
- counselling and teaching skills and techniques
- information management
- handling the mass media.

Organizational structure and processes

The student should examine factors that influence nursing practice, including:

- health care systems and the provision of health and social services
- legal frameworks
- the politics of health
- organizational structures
- management theories and trends and their application to nursing
- information systems
- national and district health and social policies.

Professional, ethical and moral issues in nursing

These issues include:

- the history and development of nursing
- autonomy, responsibility and accountability
- decision-making
- relationships with other professional groups
- concepts, principles and traditions of moral thinking
- ethical codes and moral dilemmas in nursing
- discipline and the disciplinary process
- industrial relations
- the rights of individuals, families and communities
- confidentiality, advocacy and legal responsibilities
- the role of professional statutory or licensing bodies.

5

Preparing
for leadership

Effective leadership is a key factor in motivating people, bringing about change and maintaining morale. Natural leaders emerge within most groups, but leadership qualities can also be developed.

Issues and Skills

Leadership is of crucial importance in the creation of the nurse's new role. Leaders need to be identified and supported throughout the health care system, particularly at the local or district level. Workshops on leadership can contribute to the development of leaders, organized at the interregional, regional or national levels, and useful technical advice and guidelines are already available.

Strong leadership is required at the national level, not only to encourage the development of leaders at other levels but also to emphasize and support the role of nurses in bringing about change. A valuable initiative in many countries would be the bringing together at the national level of a group of nurses who have already achieved recognition as leaders at various levels in the health system, who have influence and the confidence of their colleagues, and who have a network through which to communicate at both national and international levels. The positions of the nurses meeting such criteria will differ between countries, but such people are easily identified.

The tasks of this leadership group include initiating, planning, supporting and monitoring activities and outcomes in the development of the primary health care approach. As the group members work together, other potential leaders will emerge and begin to provide leadership in their communities. People already qualified in public health nursing and practising in peripheral areas could play an important part in the community *(40)*.

If nurse leaders are to become visible, they will have to move out and establish a variety of channels for communication with other professionals and the general public. Most leaders in nursing still tend to communicate only with others like them at meetings of nurses, through writing for professional journals or when debating nursing issues.

The obvious priority is to educate such existing nurse leaders as:

– the chiefs or directors of nursing services in ministries of health or health care institutions;

. – the heads, deans and directors of nursing schools, particularly those preparing teachers and administrators;

– the editors of nursing publications;

– major officers of nursing and nursing-related organizations;

– influential nurses involved in drawing up regulations for nursing education and practice.

These leaders' support can be enlisted and their approach changed faster than changes can be made in the curriculum for basic education. Such action will have an immediate effect on policy.

Nurses should be able to use effective strategies to manage situations and present their point of view. Techniques such as building and using networks, creating alliances, and negotiating and managing conflict and confrontation should become part of the armoury of every nurse leader. Education in these skills should take place in a variety of settings – during educational courses, through in-service training, in workshops, in political activities, in work with legislative committees and professional associations, and in the community. Developing communication skills and learning to use all forms of communication technology (television and radio, as well as newspapers and magazines) are another important source of influence.

Nurses should feel confident in leadership. The skills to achieve this can be acquired in various ways, and may mean initiating innovative modes of care delivery and then following up with evaluation (see Chapter 2). The ramifications of such assessments involve local politicians, budgets and high-profile public reaction – all essential areas in leadership development.

A critical factor is how to lead without alienating. A leader needs to be a model for other potential leaders, particularly in relation to health for all and primary health care issues; guiding others is the other half of the skill. To some this comes naturally, but both present and future nurse leaders should learn this skill. Workshops should include information on the personal and professional advantages of the activity, as well as offering instruction techniques for guiding others.

Other components of continuing education for today's nurse teachers and managers need to be developed to meet the circumstances of each country. Most will probably include the discussion of experiences in working for health for all in particular settings, as well as opportunities to develop skills necessary for effective work in groups.

Not all nursing leaders will be convinced of the need for change. At first, therefore, nurses should be carefully selected to form a core leadership, so that they may act as catalysts and involve others as they, too, become convinced.

Preparation of Nurse Teachers

In the past, the possession of technical competence and professional experience was assumed to be synonymous with an ability to teach, but the importance of learning the skills and art of teaching is now more fully appreciated. Genuine teaching experience in a postbasic programme is essential for the development of skills and confidence. The Council of Europe *(41)* recommends that nurse teachers have "advanced knowledge of sciences on which nursing is based" and states:

> c. Should teaching focus on a specialised area, e.g. community nursing or geriatric nursing, the candidate must be qualified within that field.
> d. Professional experience within the appropriate field would be required so that teaching may be seen as valid.

The skills required of nurse teachers must stress their role as facilitators of learning at all levels of the health system. For example, teachers must have a full knowledge of and commitment to the new mission and functions of the nurse (see Chapter 1) in order to reflect them in the design and implementation of curriculum changes in basic, postbasic and continuing nursing education programmes.

Teachers should also be able to adopt new approaches in planning, implementing and evaluating educational programmes at all levels. The development of such programmes will require practical skills and the provision of innovative teaching and learning experiences in a variety of settings, particularly in the community. The team approach essential to the development of primary health care will require the teacher to be able to assess the role and functions of individual team members, to understand and implement alternative methods of teamwork, to facilitate the development of leaders at all levels of the health system and, not least important, to work with people in other development sectors.

In developing innovative approaches, teachers will need to be able to prepare, use and evaluate a variety of learning aids in conducting and disseminating educational research. Teachers must also be able to build on the previous experience of their students so that learning becomes a continuous process. Teaching will thus become focused on the learner and the production of action-oriented graduates. These competences contain several levels of intellectual skill and expertise. Additional training and education are necessary for leadership in education and research.

Preparation of Nurse Managers

The abilities required of a nurse manager are largely determined by the components of the management process and the level at which the manager operates: national, intermediate or regional, local or district, or hospital. While the components are common to all levels, their relative weight will differ between levels, as will the managerial function. For example, managers at the national level need in-depth knowledge of management theory and wide managerial experience, as well as the ability to operate effectively as a member of a multiprofessional and multisectoral team. The nurse manager at the local or district level must also have this teamwork skill.

In 1989, the International Council of Nurses adopted a declaration of principle on nursing management *(42)*, regarding nurses as managers, "not merely of nurses and nursing services, but also of the health services of the future".

At the first level of management (the care unit, service or sector) the nursing manager is responsible for managing nursing care to meet the needs of patients or users. At the European Conference on Nursing in 1988, nursing managers were urged to base nursing care on the health needs and participation of the population, and to take account of:

- demographic and epidemiological trends
- the physical and social environment
- lifestyle problems
- cultural values, beliefs and ethical considerations
- economic choices and options
- the availability of qualified staff.

To do her work, the nursing manager must be competent in clinical care, to ensure optimal quality and proper management, and enjoy the professional freedom of action to allocate resources and to select, guide and train her team within the unit, service or sector.

At the intermediate level of management, the nurse manager helps to define the health care establishment's policy on care in coordination with administrative personnel and doctors, organizing and guiding the delivery of health care in the light of the available human and material resources. At the upper level of management, the nurse manager helps to design and plan health policies and participates in organizing health service delivery. She ensures that nursing care develops in ways that meet the health needs of the population as a whole.

At each of these levels the nurse manager, in addition to leadership functions in nursing care, may develop an advisory role on professional matters and be a spokesperson on all questions related to care. She should be able to formulate policies, to translate them into programmes, to make budgets, to produce and implement action plans, to determine management and organizational systems, to maintain financial controls, to monitor progress, to evaluate outcomes and to feed results back into the planning cycle.

The manager can develop these abilities through experience, provided she has a sound knowledge base. Nevertheless, a system of continuing education is necessary to sustain this development. The manager who has demonstrated competence at the local level requires additional education to prepare for the extended management role at the intermediate level.

Nurses who are to work at the national level require further education in management. This will be most relevant and efficacious if it is undertaken along with managers of other professions with whom they will subsequently work.

Postbasic Nursing Education

It is neither appropriate nor feasible to produce a blueprint for educational programmes for nurse managers and teachers. These should be developed by the competent authorities, whose first task should be to define the competences that students need to meet the health needs of the population and the requirements of a health system based on primary health care. These competences should form the basis of the objectives of postbasic education and of curriculum content.

In the context of primary health care, such objectives should not only guide action but also provide a philosophy that permeates the whole of the nursing contribution to the health care system. Postbasic education should produce graduates who can:

(a) introduce as rapidly as possible the concepts and practices of primary health care into all components of nursing education and practice;

(b) take part in the planning, management and monitoring of patterns of health care appropriate to the demographic, socioeconomic, educational, cultural, epidemiological and health service circumstances of the country;

(c) take part in the making of health policy at all levels, including priority setting, resource allocation and decision-making on action;

(d) help to achieve a more rational balance in health care, particularly in the planning, production and use of nursing personnel to provide essential, accessible and acceptable health care that meets the needs of the population;

(e) plan, implement and evaluate basic and continuing education for a variety of nursing personnel, using not only effective conventional techniques but also new strategies for teaching and learning more suited to primary health care;

(f) accelerate coordination between various components and services in the health sector to increase the effectiveness of plans for the development of human and material resources;

(g) accelerate the coordination of the health sector with other development sectors, such as those for education, housing, agriculture, social welfare, community development and public works;

(h) take part in research on the development and management of health personnel and health services, as a contribution to the emergence of further innovative patterns for primary health care development; and

(i) work as partners with communities to develop viable and effective strategies, plans and mechanisms to promote increased self-care and self-reliance.

The educational approaches and practices that nurses encounter influence their future performance and attitudes as teachers and managers. Team-based and action-oriented educational approaches are of particular relevance here. For example, participatory methods of teaching and learning are more in accord with the adult status of the students than methods that differentiate rigidly between teacher and student. The principles and practices of adult education stress creating an atmosphere of mutual learning, and this should be the aim of postbasic schools. The education principles discussed in Chapter 4 are equally relevant here.

Content of programmes

The content of postbasic educational programmes must be based in part on research. Nurse teachers and nurse managers will need to acquire knowledge of the latest epidemiological, demographic, social and economic trends. Considerable emphasis should also be placed on developing traits that negate current stereotypes of women. Thus assertiveness, risk taking, independence and self-confidence should be presented as desirable and necessary for nursing leadership. Reviews of the history of nursing, the lives of effective leaders in the profession, and literature on women's successes in achieving social change should also be included.

In many countries, nursing education and practice are controlled by authorities outside the profession. Nurses need basic knowledge of how to reach positions from which they can exercise authority and change the system in which they work. Students, managers, teachers and researchers – indeed all nurses – should therefore learn the use of systems theories as well as influence to achieve their goals.

Postbasic education should aim to develop a research mentality in students: a keen interest in continually analysing and learning from experience, an understanding of the importance of regular assessment as an integral component of their work, and an awareness of the need to develop sound information systems. Teachers must be able to assist students in learning the basic approaches to and methods of research and information collection that are relevant to important health problems and their solution. Such health service research requires that all health personnel be able to provide information about their activities; this in turn may require that they be assisted to select and collate such information. Postbasic programmes also need to prepare some researchers to conduct or direct investigations into particular primary health care issues and to undertake systematic inquiries about nursing practice. Research activities, including the systematic collection of valid information, have considerable relevance to various aspects of the management function. The ability to identify needs and to initiate or carry out the required activities is essential for good management practice; valid information is an important tool.

All nurse teachers and nurse managers should receive their professional preparation from institutes of higher education whose primary purpose is education, not service. The community outside the hospital world – with all its problems, facilities, possibilities and resources – should become the major and most frequently used location in which such nurses learn and practise their art.

Nurses must have the ability to discuss broad issues affecting health and development, if others are to listen to them. Society's growing interest in concerns relating to women gives nurses an excellent opportunity to lead such discussions from the high ground, precisely because they are experts from a predominantly female profession.

Education programmes should be assessed and restructured in the context of comprehensive national policies and plans for health personnel development. This inevitably means seeking out hidden talent and encouraging active leadership. Training centres should be identified that have the staff and facilities to create links with individuals, institutions and organizations to form resource and support networks at the national, regional and interregional levels.

The effective reorientation of postbasic nursing educational curricula will require substantive changes in the direction of policy on education, and the attitudes and values of the directors, administrators, teachers and students of postbasic education. Facilitating this process depends heavily on the ability of staff and administrators to motivate and to set an example.

One useful approach is to encourage the directors and administrators of programmes for nurse teachers and nurse managers, along with practising nurses, to investigate the health status of the community. Such direct experience will also provide information about the availability, accessibility and functioning of health services, and help create a realistic appreciation of the urgent need to make nursing education more relevant to health care needs.

It may be useful to develop countrywide networks of postbasic nursing education programmes, including those with a common concern for appropriate training for nurse teachers and managers. The members of such a network could collaborate on the use of human and material resources, and link their training programmes to facilitate development. They would be able to learn from joint ventures, to improve existing programmes, to establish new ones and to become increasingly self-reliant. Collaborative activities might include curriculum design, the preparation of teaching materials, the development of better teaching approaches, practices and appropriate methods of assessment, the sharing or exchange of learning facilities and resources, the identification of research topics and joint research ventures, and the exchange of teachers and students.

The resource requirements for the development or reorientation of postbasic education will vary from place to place. Most postbasic schools need more and better prepared teaching and support staff, training facilities and materials and educational technology. In some countries, it is difficult to obtain even the most basic equipment and supplies, such as blackboards, chalk and paper.

Many suitable educational materials exist, but institutions are often unaware of them. Where materials are obtained, adapting them may be difficult; this applies both to printed and to audiovisual aids. There is an urgent need to prepare teachers to combat these problems by producing appropriate educational technology, at low cost, from locally available materials. Experience in some countries has demonstrated that teachers and students can develop considerable skills in this area, in addition to the ability to analyse materials and to improve them after field testing.

Administrative support is crucial to the change process, and all efforts to achieve change are likely to be frustrated unless informed and committed administrators give such support. Administrators play a key role in both obtaining and allocating resources. Many countries currently face a shortage of resources for health development in general and for the reorientation required to hasten the development of primary health care in particular. In this context, postbasic schools will need to evolve relevant and cost-effective patterns of training. The ability to do this, however, will often depend on the provision of some additional resources, at least at first, and these will only become available with the support of administrators committed to change.

Steps towards improving postbasic nursing education

The following steps are given as a guide for Member States. They are neither prescriptive nor exhaustive.

1. Action should be taken to change education policies and the policies of relevant bodies (such as medical and pharmaceutical associations) that constrain the development or reorientation of nursing education programmes at all levels.

2. Action should be taken to make any changes needed in legislation or statutory requirements for nursing education and practice.

3. All postbasic education programmes for nurse teachers and managers should be reoriented to make the principles of health for all a unifying frame of reference by:

- providing short courses to reorient the directors and teachers of postbasic nursing schools and programmes;

- convening a small group of nursing leaders at the national level, made up of those who have demonstrated leadership ability at different levels in the health system, to act as a catalyst and to plan, initiate, support and monitor the reorientation;

- establishing a system of continuing education to ensure that the people who manage and teach in educational institutions and practice areas not only keep their knowledge and skills up to date, but also acquire new and deeper knowledge of the art and science of nursing;

- taking action to increase the number of qualified teachers with field experience in primary health care to assist in the reorientation and in the preparation of relevant curricula;

- identifying the competences that nurse teachers and managers need to meet the health needs of communities, and use these as a basis for defining learning objectives; and

- facilitating the achievement of the learning objectives by providing experiences that are based in and focused on the community, with community participation.

4. Problem-based, practice-oriented, team-focused, multiprofessional and multisectoral educational processes should be developed by:

- encouraging a problem-solving approach in students and giving them learning experiences in exercises and actual situations;

- using facilities such as hospitals, as well as primary health care centres and outpatient centres, to enable students to gain experience with a variety of health and other community workers; and

- providing opportunities for students to gain experience in multiprofessional and multisectoral teams in community settings.

5. Postbasic institutions and schools of nursing should be strengthened by providing needed resources and administrative support through:

- adjusting resource allocations to ensure that institutions have the human and material resources essential for programme reorientation;

- encouraging administrators to take a positive attitude towards postbasic education as the key to the development of nursing personnel;

- encouraging people in the influential hospital sector to support postbasic programmes in focusing on the community; and

- supporting the establishment of links between postbasic schools, health services and educational institutions, and the development of networks of postbasic schools for collaboration on the use of resources, the sharing of knowledge and experience, and joint endeavours.

References

1. *European Conference on Nursing.* Copenhagen, WHO Regional Office for Europe, 1989.
2. *Primary health care. Alma-Ata, 1978.* Geneva, World Health Organization, 1978 ("Health for All" Series, No. 1).
3. *Global strategy for health for all by the year 2000.* Geneva, World Health Organization, 1981 ("Health for All" Series, No. 3).
4. *Targets for health for all.* Copenhagen, WHO Regional Office for Europe, 1985 (European Health for All Series, No. 1).
5. *People's needs for nursing care: a European study.* Copenhagen, WHO Regional Office for Europe, 1987.
6. Recommendation 157 concerning employment and conditions of work and life for nursing personnel (1977). *International labour conventions and recommendations, 1919–1981.* Geneva, International Labour Office, 1986.
7. TOFFLER, A. *Future shock.* London, Pan, 1973.
8. MARTIN, J.P. *Hospitals in trouble.* London, Blackwell, 1984.
9. WRIGHT, S.G. *Changing nursing practice.* London, Edward Arnold, 1989.
10. LANCASTER, J. & LANCASTER, W. *The nurse as change agent.* St Louis, MO, Mosby, 1982.
11. PEARSON, A., ED. *Primary nursing.* London, Croom Helm, 1988.
12. OTTOWAY, R.N. A change strategy to implement new norms, new styles and new environment in the work organization. *Personnel review*, **5**(1): 13–18 (1976).
13. ROGERS, E.M. *Diffusion of innovations.* New York, Free Press, 1962.
14. KEYSER, D. Meeting the challenge. *In:* Wright, S.G. *Changing nursing practice.* London, Edward Arnold, 1989.
15. SPURGEON, P. & BARWELL, F. *Implementing change in the NHS.* London, Chapman & Hall, 1991.

111

16. *Nursing practice demonstration projects for the "generalist nurse"*. Copenhagen, WHO Regional Office for Europe, 1990 (unpublished document EUR/ICP/HSR 341).

17. MANTHEY, M. *The practice of primary nursing*. London, Blackwell, 1980.

18. *Report on the regulation of nursing*. Geneva, International Council of Nurses, 1985.

19. PEPLAU, H.E. Internal vs. external regulation. *In: Credentialing in nursing: contemporary developments and trends*. Kansas City, KA, American Nurses' Association, 1986.

20. STOREY, M. ET AL. *Guidelines for regulatory changes in nursing practice to promote primary health care*. Geneva, World Health Organization, 1988 (document WHO/EUD/88.194).

21. *Development of standards for nursing education and practice: guidelines for national nurses' associations*. Geneva, International Council of Nurses, 1989.

22. *A guide to curriculum review for basic nursing education*. Geneva, World Health Organization, 1985.

23. *European agreement on the instruction and education of nurses. Strasbourg, 25.X.1967*. Strasbourg, Council of Europe, 1978 (European Treaty Series, No. 59).

24. COMMISSION OF THE EUROPEAN COMMUNITIES. Council Directive of 27 June 1977, 77/453/EEC on Nurses. *Official journal of the European Communities*, L 176 (1977).

25. *Health for all targets: the health policy for Europe*. Copenhagen, WHO Regional Office for Europe, 1993 (European Health for All Series, No. 4).

26. *Evaluation of reoriented curricula in basic nursing education*. Geneva, World Health Organization, 1989 (document HMD/NUR 89.2).

27. *Curriculum development for the "generalist nurse"*: report on a WHO Consultation. Copenhagen, WHO Regional Office for Europe, 1990 (document EUR/ICP/HSR 340).

28. MCMURRAY, A. *Community health nursing. Primary health care in practice*. Edinburgh, Churchill Livingstone, 1990.

29. LANARA, V. *Nursing education in the 21st century. Proceedings of a symposium*. Brussels, Commission of the European Communities, 1989 (EUR 12040).

30. *Credit accumulation and transfer scheme (CATS) regulations*, 2nd ed. London, Council for National Academic Awards, 1989.

31. ROPER, N. ET AL. *The elements of nursing.* Edinburgh, Churchill Livingstone, 1985.
32. HENDERSON, V. *Basic principles of nursing care.* Geneva, International Council of Nurses, 1960.
33. *Integration of a model health component in general nursing education.* Geneva, World Health Organization, 1990.
34. WHO Technical Report Series, No. 746, 1987 *(Community-based education of health personnel).*
35. *Managing change in nursing education. Pack 1.* London, English National Board for Nursing, Midwifery and Health Visiting, 1988.
36. BRADSHAW, P.L. *Teaching and assessing in nursing practice.* Englewood Cliffs, NJ, Prentice-Hall, 1989.
37. DEPARTMENT OF HEALTH AND NURSING STUDIES, GLASGOW POYTECHNIC. *Course document for BA (Hons) degree in nursing studies.* Glasgow, Glasgow Polytechnic, 1990.
38. ALLAN, P. & JOLLEY, M. *The curriculum in nursing education.* London, Chapman & Hall, 1987.
39. PARLETT, M. & HAMILTON, D. *Evaluation as illumination.* Edinburgh, Centre for Research in the Educational Sciences, Edinburgh University, 1972 (Occasional Paper No. 9).
40. WHO Technical Report Series, No. 708, 1984 (*Education and training of nurse teachers and managers with special regard to primary health care:* report of a WHO Expert Committee).
41. *Further training for nurses in the member states of the Council of Europe and in Finland.* Strasbourg, Council of Europe, 1983.
42. *Guidelines for national nursing associations and others. Preparation of nurse managers and nurses in general health management.* Geneva, International Council of Nurses, 1991.

Recommendations from the European Conference on Nursing

1. All nurses, their professional associations, nongovernmental organizations and volunteer groups should be strong advocates for policies and programmes for health for all at national, regional and local levels.

2. Innovative nursing services should be developed that focus on health rather than disease; patterns of work should be appropriate, efficient and conducive to primary health care. Governments, health authorities and nurses' professional organizations should take urgent steps to remove factors that inhibit this process and should draw up or modify legislation and regulations to ensure that nurses are able to meet their responsibilities as front-line workers in primary health care.

3. In keeping with European policies for health for all, the nurse's practice should be based mainly on the principles inherent in the primary health care approach. The focus should be on:

- promoting and maintaining health, and preventing disease;

- involving individuals, families and communities in care and making it possible for them to take more responsibility for their health;

- working actively to reduce inequities in access to health care services and to satisfy the needs of whole populations, especially the underserved;

- multidisciplinary and multisectoral collaboration; and

- assurance of the quality of care and the appropriate use of technology.

4. All basic programmes of nursing education should be restructured, reoriented and strengthened, in order to produce generalist nurses able to function in both hospital and community. All specialist knowledge and skills subsequently acquired should be built on this foundation. Nursing education should include ample experience outside the hospital. Candidates for nursing education should have completed a full secondary education (which may vary from country to country) and have qualifications for admission that are equivalent to those required by a university or other institute of higher education. The directors of schools of nursing or departments of nursing education, and teachers and supervisors of nursing programmes must all be nurses.

5. Nurses managing care and services must base care on the health needs and participation of the population, in accordance with the regional strategy for health for all, and must take account of:

- demographic and epidemiological trends
- the social and physical environment
- lifestyle issues
- cultural values and beliefs and ethical considerations
- economic choices and alternatives
- the qualified personnel available.

Nurse managers must have professional autonomy, so that they can allocate resources in accordance with the principles of the health for all strategy.

6. To ensure the full cooperation of the nursing community, nurse researchers should be appointed to all national research councils dealing with health or related research, including bodies such as the WHO European Advisory Committee on Health Research.

WHO should urge nurses to start community care demonstration projects that produce measurable improvements in care and promote the efficient use of resources in selected communities.

To permit the development of community-oriented nursing practice, education and leadership, nursing research must be a part of all fields of practice.

An equitable share of existing funds should be made available for nursing research projects.

7. WHO, its collaborating centres, intergovernmental and non-governmental organizations, and national nurses' associations should set up information systems and increase communication and the dissemination of information and research results through national, regional and international networks. Modern technology should be used to strengthen links between consumer and other groups, organizations and institutes.

8. Nursing should be included as one of the essential elements of national health plans now being developed, based on the regional strategy for health for all, and nurses should take part in the debate on health policy.

Legislation on nursing practice should recognize the nurse's contribution to the organization, development and delivery of health care. It should be formulated in a way that promotes nurses' ability to meet the health needs of the population.

9. In the light of demographic trends and their implications for the development of primary health care, health manpower policies should be based on health for all and should include:

- a plan to recruit nursing personnel, drawn up in collaboration with nurses, administrators and politicians and using current manpower databases;

- terms and conditions of service that attract and retain qualified nurses, ensure the appropriate use of nursing personnel, and recognize continuing education as part of career development;

- a programme of continuing education accessible to all nurses;

- counselling programmes for personal and career development.

10. In view of nurses' strong influence as role models for the population, individual nurses and nurses' organizations have a special responsibility to exemplify a healthy lifestyle and, more specifically, to support the concerted European action against tobacco by promoting smoke-free working environments. Cessation counselling should be made available to all nurses who smoke.

Vienna Declaration on Nursing in Support of the European Targets for Health for All

The participants at the European Conference on Nursing, meeting in Vienna from 21 to 24 June 1988, express the need for urgent action by governments and national health decision-makers to help nurses make the changes that are required in nursing if the regional targets for health for all are to be achieved, and hereby make the following declaration:

I

Health, which is a state of complete physical, mental and social wellbeing and not merely the absence of disease or infirmity, is a fundamental human right. The attainment of the highest possible level of health is a most important social goal, whose realization requires the action of many professions.

II

The persisting inequalities in people's health status, both between and within countries of the WHO European Region, are politically, socially, economically and professionally unacceptable and are therefore of common concern to all nurses.

III

Having provided nurses from the 32 countries in the Region with their first opportunity to re-examine their role, education and practice, the

Conference reaffirms the status of nursing as a force that can make a major contribution to achieving the 38 targets adopted by the Member States at the thirty-fourth session of the WHO Regional Committee for Europe in 1984.

IV

The participants pledge to bring the new role of the nurse in the era of health for all to the attention of ministries of health, the organizations and trade unions of all health professions, regulatory bodies and other groups throughout the Region. Nurses should develop their new role by: acting as partners in decision-making on the planning and management of local, regional and national health services; playing a greater role in empowering individuals, families and communities to become more self-reliant and to take charge of their health development; and providing clear and valid information on the favourable and adverse consequences of various types of behaviour, and on the merits and costs of different options for care.

V

New attitudes and values need to be fostered among all health professionals, health care consumers and related groups that are consistent with the directives and principles of health for all and the primary health care approach. Nursing can best fulfil its potential in primary health care when nursing education provides a sound foundation for nursing practice, especially work in the community, and when nurses take account of the social aspects of health needs and have a broader understanding of health development. Policies should be adopted and activities identified to enable nurses to practise with sufficient autonomy to carry out their new role in primary health care.

VI

Research to improve nursing practice along these lines should be encouraged through the creation of research policies and financial support. Such research should use human resources efficiently, and ensure the evaluation and use of its results. Nurses should also be involved in the research process.

Resolution WHA45.5 of the Forty-fifth World Health Assembly on strengthening nursing and midwifery in support of strategies for health for all, May 1992

The Forty-fifth World Health Assembly,

Having considered the Director-General's report on strengthening nursing and midwifery in support of strategies for health for all, and the discussions at the eigthty-ninth session of the Executive Board;

Recalling resolution WHA42.27;

Mindful of the growing demand for and cost of health care in countries throughout the world;

Concerned at the continued shortage of nursing and midwifery pesonnel and the urgent need to recruit, retain, educate and motivate sufficient numbers to meet present and future community health needs;

Recognizing the need to increase the Organization's nursing and midwifery activities at all levels;

Committed to the promotion of nursing and midwifery as essential health services in all countries, for the development and improvement of health-for-all strategies;

1. THANKS the Director-General for his report;

2. URGES Member States to:

    (1)   identify their nursing and midwifery service needs and, in this context, assess the roles and utilization of nursing and midwifery personnel;

    (2)   strengthen managerial and leadership capabilities and reinforce the positions of nursing and midwifery personnel in all health care settings and at all levels of service, including the central and local services of health ministries and the local authorities responsible for the programmes concerned;

    (3)   enact legislation, where necessary, or take other appropriate measures to ensure good nursing and midwifery services;

    (4)   strengthen education in nursing and midwifery, adapt educational programmes to the strategy for health for all, and revise them where appropriate, in order to meet the changing health care needs of populations;

    (5)   promote and support health services research that will ensure the optimal contribution of nursing and midwifery to health care delivery, with particular emphasis on primary health care;

    (6)   ensure appropriate working conditions in order to sustain the motivation of personnel and improve the quality of services;

    (7)   ensure the allocation of adequate resources (financial, human and logistic) for nursing and midwifery activities;

    (8)   ensure that the contribution of nursing and midwifery is reflected in health policies;

3. REQUESTS WHO regional committees to reinforce regional actions in order to enable Member States to implement the above provisions effectively and to identify sources for financing such actions in those States which are undergoing economic structural reform programmes or which have other special needs;

4. REQUESTS the Director-General to:

(1) establish a global multidisciplinary advisory group on nursing and midwifery, with the express purpose of advising the Director-General on all nursing and midwifery services and in particular on:

(a) developing mechanisms for assessing national nursing and midwifery service needs;

(b) assisting countries with the development of national action plans for nursing and midwifery services including research and resource planning;

(c) monitoring progress in strengthening nursing and midwifery in support of strategies for health for all;

(2) mobilize the increased technical and financial support required to implement the provisions of this resolution;

(3) ensure that the interests of nursing and midwifery services are taken into account in policy implementation and programme development, and that nursing and midwifery experts participate in WHO committees as appropriate;

(4) strengthen the global network of WHO collaborating centres for nursing and midwifery in the implementation of health for all;

(5) report on progress made in the implementation of this resolution to the Forty-ninth World Health Assembly.